Exploring Herbal Approaches for Heart-Health

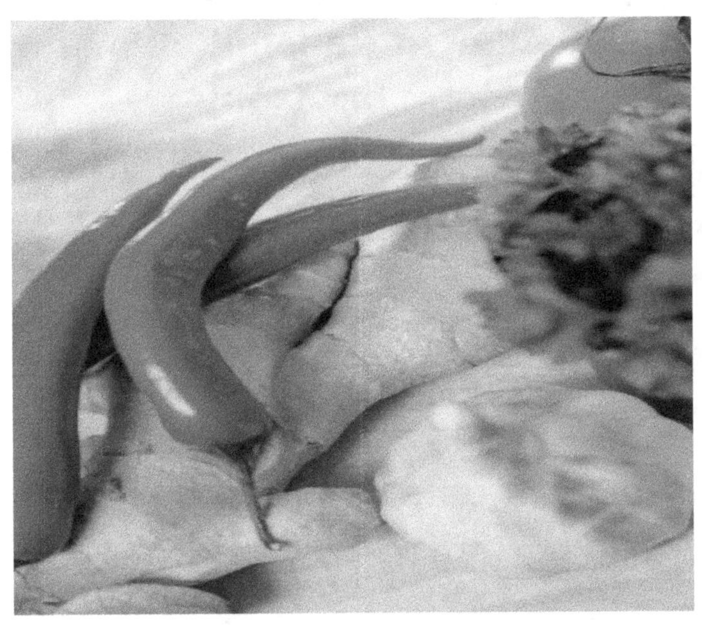

Harmonizing Heart by Nurturing Wellness Through Herbal Pathways

Shamika L. Braden

TABLE OF CONTENTS

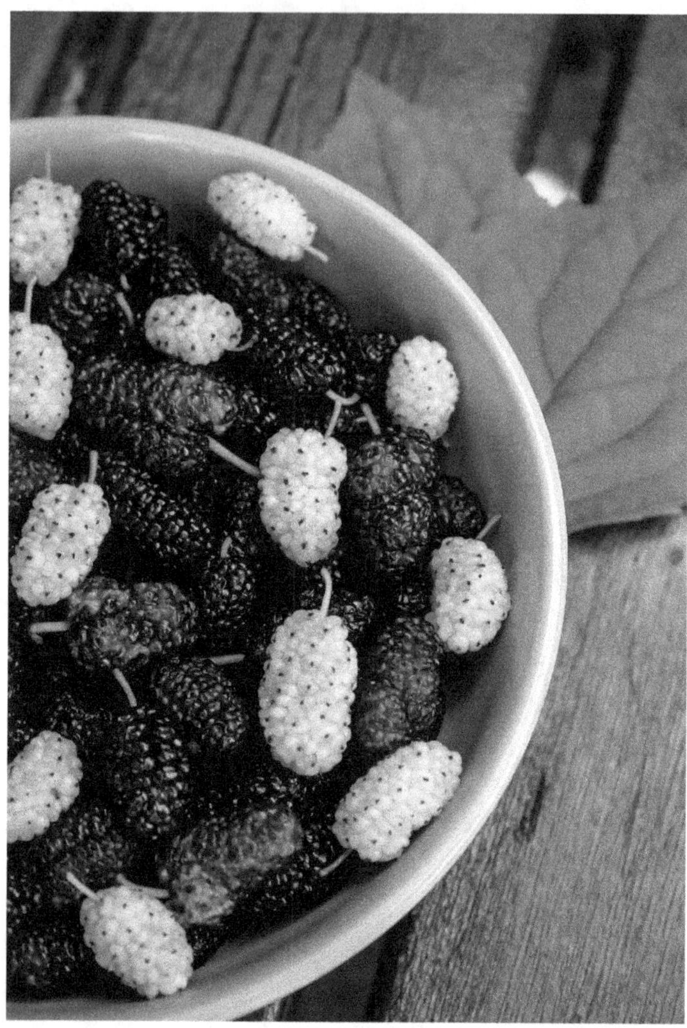

PREFACE

Our hearts beat as the rhythmic conductors of our lives, keeping us in touch with the outside world as we travel through life. Our fragile yet strong hearts are the key to our well-being, guiding each action we take. We find ourselves at a crossroads where current knowledge and time-tested methods combine, at the nexus of contemporary medical achievements and ancient wisdom.

Exploring Herbal Approaches for Heart-Health explores the pathways of holistic well-being with an emphasis on the heart, the physical manifestation of life itself. In this guide, ancient allies given to us by the earth's bounty, herbs, smoothly meld with cutting-edge knowledge to provide a peaceful route to promoting heart-health.

Do you or a loved one struggle with heart-related conditions? The value of preventative treatment cannot be overemphasized in a society where heart-related issues are becoming a factor in doctor visits and hospital admissions. Worldwide, cardiovascular disease has a devastating impact on millions of people, leading us to look for alternatives to protect the health of our hearts.

A lot of information is included within these pages, illuminating the field of heart-health from a viewpoint that combines time-tested methods with cutting-edge expertise. Its fundamental tenet is the knowledge that, while medical intervention is essential, a holistic strategy may effortlessly support traditional approaches, boosting the complex symphony of our cardiovascular system.

A harmonious partnership between science and the environment is beneficial for heart-health. We may rely on a symposium of herbs—those amazing partners the earth has so generously given us—to promote the health of our circulatory system. When used carefully and wisely, these botanical marvels may support sensible lifestyle changes and provide a holistic plan to maintain the vitality of our hearts.

As an organ and a representation, the heart captures the essence of life by vibrating with energy and resonating with emotions. You will come across a tapestry of herbs as you flip the pages that follow; each thread has been woven with care and purpose, and together they create a mosaic that supports heart-health. Throughout your investigation, you will come across a collection of plants that can nourish the vibrancy of our hearts, and each one carries the whispers of previous generations as well as the power to influence future generations.

"Exploring Herbal Approaches for Heart-Health" encourages you to accept the synthesis of conventional knowledge and timeless knowledge. It provides knowledge, direction, and a path to a heart-centered way of living where the resonance of herbs meets the beat of life. Enter a world where human curiosity and nature's medicines work together to promote a heartbeat that is healthier and more energetic.

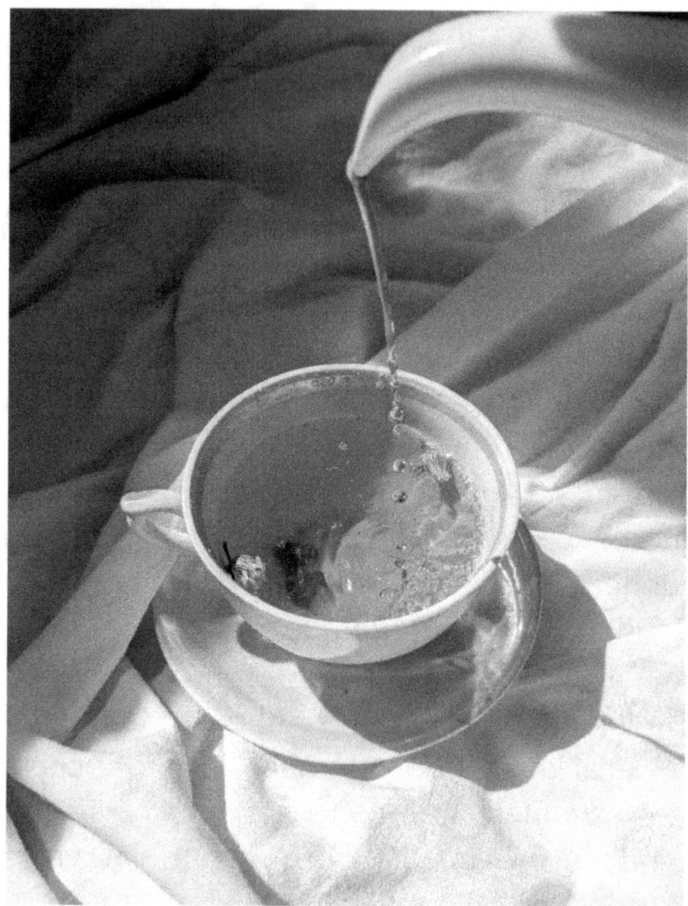

<u>INTRODUCTION</u>

I went to the doctor around 17 years ago because I had a urinary tract infection. But to my amazement, the nurse's normal examination of my vital signs revealed that my blood pressure was shockingly high at 176/121. The doctor expressed clear worry and even considered checking me into the hospital. I politely declined, thinking of my wise great-grandma's advice to "stay out of the hospital," which she had frequently repeated throughout her almost 100-year life. In there, they'll murder you. This remark resonated with me, probably as a result of my early employment in a hospital's cardiology department, where I did EKGs on patients and saw more than I felt comfortable seeing in other medical departments.

Please be aware that I am not against proper medical treatment. I am aware that some circumstances call for medical attention. My preference, however, has grown more toward a holistic strategy as a result of my familiarity with herbal medicines and essential oils. I've been managing my health naturally for the past 10 years, avoiding over-the-counter and prescription drugs. Even though I now rely on herbs, essential oils, and holistic approaches for my continuous health needs, I would still seek medical assistance if I broke my leg.

Despite my resistance, the doctor urged me to take medicine to decrease my blood pressure right away on the day of the occurrence. Unfortunately, the drug made me feel sick all day. My interest in heart-health was sparked by this incident, which encouraged me to do some research.

About 17 years ago, this event signaled a turning point in my life and led me to pursue a natural health route that mostly focused on herbs. This change is a benefit, along with a few other things. Did you know that the leading cause of hospital stays and doctor visits nowadays is cardiovascular disease? Surprisingly, heart-related problems claim the lives of over 650,000 people each year, making cardiovascular disease the top cause of mortality for both men and women.

My 20-year fight with high blood pressure enhanced my path into heart-health, specifically blood pressure control. However, I've been able to get my readings into the pre-hypertensive region for diastolic readings and fairly close to normal for systolic readings. This resulted from the daily ingestion of particular herbs and the development of healthy living practices.

Many of the students in my course have achieved the same results with the personalized regimen I developed. Understanding holistic health options and figuring out which plants work best with your particular body is key.

Fewer people are aware that incorporating herbs into your daily routine can significantly improve overall heart-health, including blood pressure management. The majority are familiar with the traditional lifestyle changes that can positively influence blood pressure, such as exercise, weight management, and a balanced diet.

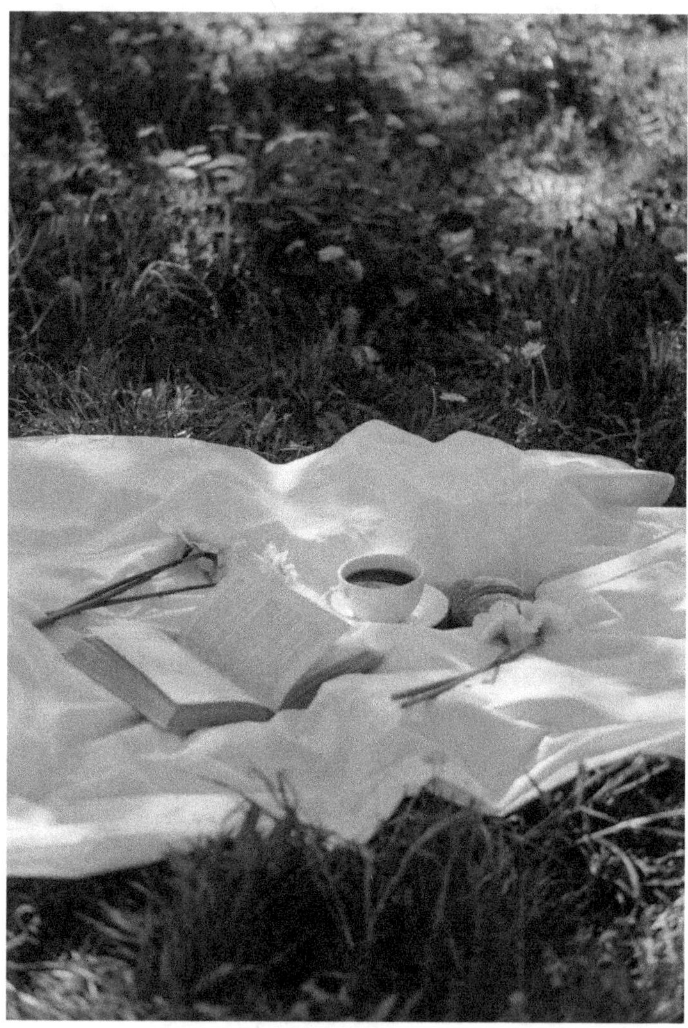

CHAPTER ONE: Unveiling the Herbal Symphony for Heart-Health

Our hearts take center stage in the complex dance of existence, arranging the beats that direct our path. They throb with purpose, balancing fragility and resiliency in a delicate dance that holds the secret to our well-being. This chapter begins an enlightening adventure as we enter the world of heart-health. It's like pulling back the curtain on a great symphony where herbs and holistic methods harmoniously coexist.

1.1 Recognizing the Connection Between Herbs and Heart Wellness

We find ourselves at a crossroads of tradition and innovation, where old wisdom and modern insight effortlessly combine in a world bursting with medical discoveries. We are on the verge of discovering a holistic approach to heart-health in these pages, a tapestry made of herbal threads, each of which has a distinctive melody in the big symphony of wellbeing.

The complex relationship between herbs and heart-health emerges as our understanding of holistic well-being grows. The comprehensive acceptance of nature's riches benefits our hearts, the beating centers of life. The botanical wonders and profound grasp of the relationships between nature and our internal rhythms are all embodied in the symphony of herbs.

This chapter serves as an introduction to the beneficial relationship between herbs and heart wellness. It's the revealing of the subtle interactions that give us the confidence and grace to go through the complex dance of life.

Synergy, in the context of heart-health, refers to the fusion of age-old wisdom with the swift advances of modern science. It is our understanding that herbs, because of their powerful powers, provide not only bodily hydration but also emotional and spiritual resonance. This synergy encourages a more profound awareness of well-being, where the heartbeat of nature harmonizes with our own.

Imagine the herbal symphony as a tapestry made of hibiscus, hawthorn, rooibos, motherwort, ginger, cayenne pepper, celery, and garlic as we enter this study. Every herb offers a different note, a different resonance, that plays a part in the unified whole of heart-health. Our hearts flourish when the symphony of herbs is performed in unison with a healthy lifestyle, just as a symphony requires the talent of numerous instruments to create a unified masterpiece.

1.2 The Echoes of Tradition and Modernity

This chapter's main idea is in line with the guide's primary goal, which is to link the past's knowledge with the present's inventions. It acts as a call to action to interact with the herbal symphony, a composition that develops over time and is a testament to the healing potential of nature in each note.

We must respect tradition and acknowledge the herbal treatments that have withstood the test of time if we are to unveil the herbal symphony. At the same time, it inspires us to accept the wonders of contemporary science and make use of knowledge that can improve the effectiveness of these time-honored traditions.

We must pay attention to both the future's rhythm and the past's whispers as we travel the path of comprehending the relationship between herbs and heart wellness. It involves accepting the knowledge of our forebears while cultivating an open-hearted openness to the potential of the unknowable.

1.3 Harmonizing Heart: An Ongoing Melody

We begin a voyage of discovery that echoes the music of our emotions as this chapter's curtain rises. We seek not just bodily well-being but also a closer relationship with the natural world and ourselves through the harmony of herbs. This investigation is a call to participate in a heart-centered, thoughtful conversation with nature's gifts.

Keep in mind that the herbal symphony is a continuous tune when we read the chapters that come after this one. It is a rhythm that permeates every aspect of our lives and directs us toward a peaceful life where the wisdom of herbs and the orchestration of well-being are used to promote heart-health.

Let's enter the heart of the symphony in the spirit of this reveal, where herbs and heart wellness combine to create a melodious path toward holistic vitality.

1.4 Navigating a Holistic Approach to Cardiovascular Care

A holistic approach serves as a guiding light, lighting a thorough journey toward cardiac well-being amid the broad expanse of healthcare options. This chapter spreads its wings within the framework of heart-health, allowing us to make our way through the maze of holistic cardiovascular care. The symphony of herbs takes center stage and resonates with the beat of our hearts in a world where medical discoveries are combined with a deep regard for old wisdom.

The concept that heart-health extends beyond the physical and affects emotional, mental, and even spiritual wellness is at the core of our investigation. The holistic approach recognizes how intertwined we all are and how the harmonic alignment of the mind, body, and spirit dances together.

Adopting a holistic approach to cardiovascular treatment means seeing the heart not as an independent structure but as a vital component of the complex ecosystem that makes up our entire well-being. It's an acknowledgment that supporting the heart necessitates a multifaceted approach going beyond traditional medical procedures.

Imagine yourself navigating through a complex tapestry of practices as we explore this chapter, including food decisions, lifestyle changes, mindfulness exercises, and the tremendous impact of herbs. Instead of being a single, linear voyage, this navigation is a dynamic, continuing process with a rhythmic cadence that beats in time with our hearts.

The holistic method encourages us to take an active role in our quest for wellness by developing a relationship with our bodies and accepting the responsibility of being aware caregivers. It's a powerful journey that gives us the information, comprehension, and tools we need to successfully navigate the currents of heart-health.

Navigating a holistic approach to cardiovascular care is essentially like setting out on a journey where each decision, each action, and each herb infusion complement the melody of our hearts. It's a journey that calls for listening to nature's guidance, respecting tradition's nudges, and accepting science's discoveries.

We'll come across the many plants that each provide a distinctive melody to the herbal symphony as we make our way deeper into the center of our excursion. The beneficial relationship between these medicines and our cardiovascular health is evidence of the complex dance of holistic health.

As you continue reading, picture yourself as a navigator, using the holistic compass to navigate through the wide sea of well-being. Every choice you make, every revelation you have, and every herb you use all ring with the vibrancy of your heart. Additionally, keep in mind that you are not alone on this journey; nature's wisdom and the synthesis of ancient and modern science serve as lighthouses, pointing you in the direction of a harmonious and all-encompassing approach to cardiovascular care.

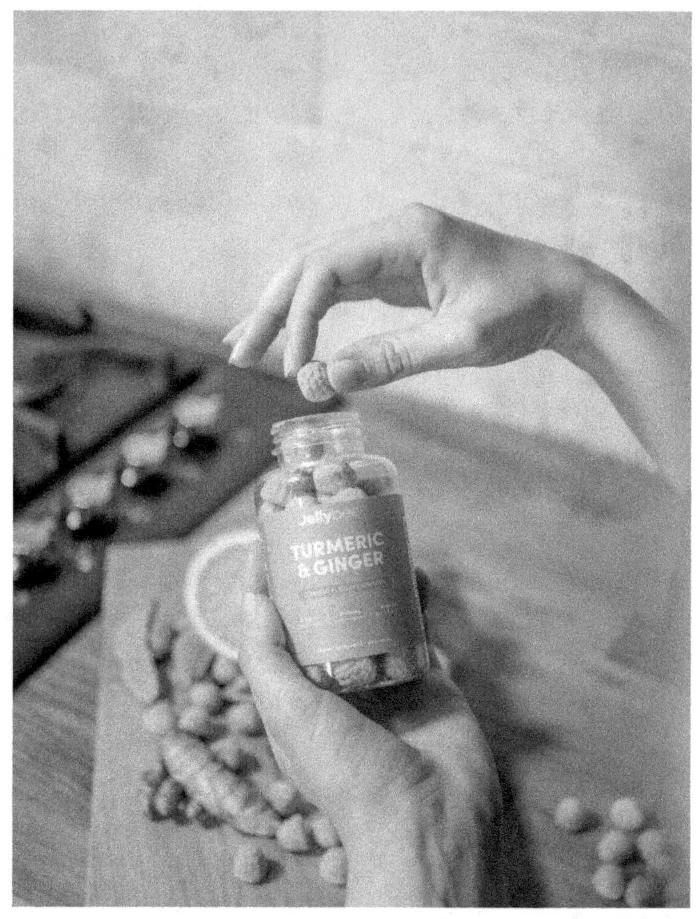
JellyCo
TURMERIC
& GINGER

CHAPTER TWO: Hibiscus: Nurturing Nature's Elixir

2.1 Hibiscus Use for heart-health

Each chapter unfolds like a melodic note in the symphony of holistic health as we go farther into the breadth of heart-centered well-being. We enter the second chapter, similar to a delicate melody in the ensemble, just as a conductor orchestrates the lovely mix of instruments: Hibiscus: Nurturing Nature's Elixir. As we examine the heart-supporting properties of hibiscus, this chapter nicely demonstrates how the holistic approach harmonizes with the principles of cardiovascular care.

The Vivid Elixir of Hibiscus Petals

Imagine a brilliant crimson tea that has been expertly brewed from hibiscus flower-dried petals. It would be a marvel in both sight and taste. This lovely plant graces civilizations all over the world with its presence and thrives in warm, frequently tropical climates. Hibiscus has etched a place in the fabric of traditions and is referred to as "Sour Tea" in Iran and "Red Sorrel" in England. It is a beloved component in many commercial tea blends thanks to its acidic but delectable flavor.

Hibiscus has more appeal than just its sweetness since it has the intrinsic ability to promote cardiovascular health. The anthocyanins, which are defensive substances that have a preference for protecting certain organs within our bodies, are what give it its beautiful red calyxes. Hibiscus enters the scene as a cardiotonic plant, supporting good blood pressure and maybe aiding in natural cholesterol control, with the health of the heart as its primary concern. This stunning plant, decorated in crimson tones, develops into more than simply a visual treat; it develops into a tonic for life.

The Heartbeat of Research

Numerous clinical studies have looked at the beneficial effects of hibiscus on heart-health. Its involvement in cardiovascular treatment is credible because of its reputation for potentially assisting in blood pressure lowering. Simply have two cups of this delicious tea every day—a soothing ritual that nurtures the heart within—to fill your routine with the advantages of hibiscus.

Beyond its importance to science, hibiscus exudes a sense of gastronomic adaptability. It is the ideal accompaniment to homemade lemonades, bringing taste and practical value due to its cooling nature and sour tone. The essence of holistic nourishment—where flavor, scent, and well-being converge—resonates with this plant, which surpasses the boundaries of traditional medicine.

Hibiscus: A Herbal Ally for the Heart

Hibiscus, which is Generally Recognized as Safe (GRAS), enters the holistic arena as a heartfelt companion. However, it is advised to speak with a healthcare provider before adding any new herbal allies to your routine in the interest of responsible wellness. This action is consistent with the underlying concept of the guide, which is that ancient knowledge may coexist peacefully with contemporary awareness.

If you're inclined to explore the scientific side of hibiscus, there are a ton of fascinating findings just waiting to be discovered. The delicate interaction between the hibiscus and the heart, enhanced by scientific intricacies, serves as a bridge between traditional devotion and contemporary validation.

As we conclude this part, keep in mind that each drink of hibiscus tea has not only its distinct flavor but also the echoes of earlier generations and the prospect of a heart that is healthier. Hibiscus is the essence of "Exploring Herbal Approaches for heart-health," resonating as a heart-nourishing note in the herbal symphony.

2.2 Ways to Include Hibiscus in Your Routine

It doesn't take major adjustments to include the bright symphony of hibiscus into your daily rhythm; rather, it begs you to enrich your routine with its wholesome essence. As you explore various hibiscus-incorporation strategies, the path to heart-health turns into a joyous adventure.

- Hibiscus Infusion: Creating a hot cup of hibiscus tea is the foundation of hibiscus integration. Watch as the water turns into a rich red elixir when you immerse the dried petals in hot water. You may drink this energizing tea unsweetened or with a little honey for sweetness.

- Refreshing Hibiscus Lemonade: Up your hydration game by adding the tart flavors of hibiscus to your traditional lemonade. For a refreshing summer beverage, combine the hibiscus tea with freshly squeezed lemon juice, a touch of sweetness, and a splash of sparkling water.

- Hibiscus exceeds the limits of drinks, as stated in Culinary Adventures. Hibiscus petals may be used in salads, dressings, and even sauces to give them a distinctive flavor. Your culinary canvas has an artistic touch from the vivid hue.

- As the temperature rises, turn your hibiscus infusion into a refreshing beverage. Iced Hibiscus Elixir Make a concentrated hibiscus tea and put it in the refrigerator. When you're thirsty, combine it with cold water, some lemon juice, and maybe some mint.

- Utilize the synergy of herbs by combining hibiscus with complementary allies. Hibiscus with herbs like ginger, rosehip, or lemongrass makes a lovely infusion. Each herb improves the qualities of the others, resulting in a delicious symphony of flavors and advantages.

- Hibiscus should be used as a little herbal flavoring in your homemade popsicles. Hibiscus tea is combined with the fruit of your choosing, then poured into molds and frozen. These cool delights offer a vibrant and beneficial approach to fighting the heat.

- Expand your hibiscus exploration beyond food with hibiscus-infused oil. By soaking the petals in a carrier oil, you can create a hibiscus-infused oil. This fragrant oil may be poured into your bath for a soothing sensory experience or used for light massages.

Hibiscus welcomes you to discover the wide range of its flavors, colors, and advantages by making it a part of your routine. Each technique is consistent with the central idea of the guide. a comprehensive strategy for heart-health that combines innovation and tradition to create a seamless fabric of well-being. Hibiscus has many benefits for your days, and while you enjoy them, you're intentionally nurturing your heart by embracing what nature has to offer.

2.3 Hibiscus and Flavorful Foods: A Culinary Companion"

In the world of cooking, the art of combining ingredients is like a symphony of tastes, where each note works in harmony to produce a masterpiece for the palate. In this culinary composition, hibiscus, with its tart and vivid personality, transforms into a flexible companion, bringing depth and complexity to a range of recipes.

- Sensational Salads: Hibiscus may take your salads to a new level. Hibiscus's acidic undertones combine with the crispness of leafy greens to create a revitalizing symphony of tastes. Hibiscus petals may be added to a salad of mixed greens to add a surprising pop of color and flavor.

- A fruity mix combines the acidity of hibiscus with the sweetness of fruits to create a delicious mix. Fruit salads, compotes, or jams will benefit from the "brilliant color and alluring flavor that dried hibiscus petals may impart.

- Hibiscus may add layers of nutritious goodness to yogurt parfaits, making them more filling and satisfying. The petals add their heart-healthy qualities to your morning routine while also adding aesthetic appeal and a tangy edge to the creamy yogurt.

- Expand your knowledge of food by incorporating hibiscus into sauces and condiments. Hibiscus' strong taste accentuates vinaigrettes, elevating everyday salads to remarkable gourmet experiences.

- Exquisite Desserts: Desserts and hibiscus go together like bread and butter. Cake mixtures, muffin mixes, or even homemade ice cream may all benefit from the enticing taste that dried hibiscus flowers provide.

- Hibiscus isn't just used to make desserts; it can also make savory foods more flavorful, according to Grilled Magic. Try making hibiscus marinades for grilled meats or veggies. The infusion adds a distinctive acidity that counteracts the grilled taste's richness.

- Combine the benefits of hibiscus with those of other herbal companions to create complex tea blends in Herbal Teas with a Twist. It may be used with chamomile to create a calming infusion or with mint to create a rejuvenating beverage.

Hibiscus may be paired with a variety of savory cuisines for an experiment in flavor, texture, and originality. As you embrace the culinary company of hibiscus, you start a journey that honors the holistic nature of heart-health, where each meal turns into a reflection of the guide's main theme: the harmony of nature's gifts with human well-being. Through this culinary journey, your meals become more than just survival food—they become an embodiment of the symphony of well-being.

2.4 Serving Up Hibiscus: Fresh and Inspiring Recipes

Hibiscus emerges as a multifaceted protagonist in the world of culinary research, adding its colorful personality to a variety of energizing and inventive foods and drinks. Hibiscus adds a surprise element to the symphony of your meals that is good for the heart's health as well as the senses.

- Hibiscus-Infused Water: Make staying hydrated a fine art by adding hibiscus flowers to your water. The end product is a visually attractive, slightly tart elixir that not only satisfies thirst but also gives your daily hydration regimen a touch of class.

- Hibiscus makes it simple to create mocktails with enticing flavors and brilliant colors, according to the guide Mocktail Magic. Create a wonderful, alcohol-free beverage by combining hibiscus tea with sparkling water, lemon juice, and honey. It's ideal for any occasion.

- A handmade hibiscus sorbet is a refreshing way to escape the heat. Hibiscus tea is combined with a little sweetness and then frozen. Enjoy spoonfuls of this refreshing, tangy treat that not only satisfies your sweet tooth but also soothes your heart.

- Hibiscus may elevate your morning smoothie routine. Floral Smoothie Fusion Hibiscus tea is combined with a variety of fruits, yogurt, and a small amount of ice to create a vivid, nutrient-rich cocktail that boosts your cardiovascular health as well as your senses.

- Hibiscus-Infused Vinegar: Infuse vinegar with hibiscus blossoms to transform your condiments. Each bite of your salads and marinades becomes a gastronomic journey that resonates with heart-health thanks to the tangy infusion that results.

- Create a hibiscus relish that dances between sweet and salty in the recipe "Sweet and Savory Relishes. For a relish that tastes amazing with grilled meats or as a dip for tortilla chips, combine hibiscus petals with chopped fruits like mango or pineapple and a dash of chile pepper.

- Start your mornings with a bowl of hibiscus-infused oats for a heart-nourishing boost. As your porridge cooks, mix hibiscus tea into it to make a hearty breakfast that reflects the holistic philosophy of the guide.

Hibiscus may be served in these inventive and revitalizing ways, expanding your culinary options and allowing the symphony of tastes to speak to your taste buds and overall well-being. You are balancing the gifts of nature with the rhythm of your heart's energy with each creative meal and beverage. As you explore these culinary horizons, keep in mind that maintaining good heart-health requires a journey that combines innovation and tradition, making each meal a satisfying and musical experience.

2.5 Timing Matters: When to Enjoy Hibiscus Benefits

Timing sets up an important rhythm in the symphony of heart-health. Knowing the best times to enjoy hibiscus' advantages is essential for maximizing their effectiveness. Consuming hibiscus at the right time, whether as a calming nightcap or a morning habit, is consistent with the holistic philosophy of the guide.

- Morning Elixir: Start the day off well with hibiscus-infused water or a vivacious hibiscus smoothie. The energizing tanginess stimulates your senses and creates a peaceful atmosphere for the hours to come.

- Midday Refreshment: Accept hibiscus as a midday dipper. Hibiscus tea has calming effects that can help your body and mind relax despite the activity of the day. Sip some during a moment of rest.

- Pre-Meal Prelude: Use hibiscus as part of your pre-meal ritual to get your body ready for food. Its capacity to promote healthy digestion complements the mindful approach to heart-health, boosting total physical and mental well-being.

- Evening Tranquility: Hibiscus assumes the role of a calming friend when the sun sets. Enjoy a cup of hibiscus tea in the evening and allow its relaxing qualities to help you ease into some peaceful moments of sleep.

The time spent enjoying hibiscus perfectly captures the central concept of the guide: cooperating with nature's guidance to preserve the health of the heart. Whether taken in the early morning or late at night, each sip resonates as a thoughtful stride towards comprehensive well-being and a harmonious embrace of the symphony of heart-health.

2.6 Dosage Guidelines: Choosing Your Ideal Hibiscus Wellness Cup

Finding the proper ingredients and knowing how much of them to consume is just the beginning of the road to heart-health. The vivid characteristics of the hibiscus also fit into this motif. While savoring its taste is delightful, getting the appropriate dosage guarantees you get the most out of it.

- Balancing Act: Moderation is key to striking a balance. As a general rule, it is frequently advised to drink two cups of hibiscus tea daily to benefit from any potential heart-supportive properties. This moderation enables your body to receive its benefits without overtaxing it.

- Individual Variations: Keep in mind that every person's body is different. Your recommended dose may vary based on your age, health, and personal responses. Pay attention to how your body reacts, and think about getting advice from a medical expert.

- Holistic Synergy: The holistic perspective of the guide invites you to take hibiscus into account as a component of a holistic routine. The dose involves more than just an amount; it also considers how hibiscus works in harmony with other heart-nourishing techniques to nourish not only your physical health but also your total well-being.

- Wellness Journey: Your road to heart wellness is a unique quest. Hibiscus doses should represent your desire to synchronize with nature's gifts as you travel this road. Each cup of hibiscus, whether it is a morning ritual or a nighttime wind-down, resonates with your dedication to preserving the vibrancy of the symphony in your heart.

CHAPTER THREE: Hawthorn Leaf and Berries: Protectors of Cardiovascular Health

3.1 Investigating Hawthorn's Potential for heart-health

As we proceed in harmony along the lanes of cardiovascular wellness. We investigate the heart-supporting properties of hawthorn—nature's keepers of cardiovascular health—much like a conductor leads a symphony. The holistic health concept resounds in this chapter as it reveals the mutually beneficial link between hawthorn and heart-health.

Hawthorn's Heart-Centric Symphony

Hawthorn reveals its complex personality through its leaves, berries, and blooms, which come together to create a heart-centered symphony of well-being. Hawthorn has great advantages for the heart due to its high flavonoid content, notably proanthocyanidin. This organic gift from the land supports the heart's rhythm and vigor and harmonizes well with the holistic spirit of the guide.

Arterial Pathway Dilation

Science has made The significant effects of hawthorn on cardiovascular health clear. Its contact with the heart mostly involves widening the arteries, a process that improves blood flow and is evidence of nature's capacity for nurturing. The concept of the guide connects with the peaceful rhythm that Hawthorn creates, showing how herbal remedies and heart-health may coexist harmoniously.

Hawthorn: A Guardian's Embrace

Hawthorn represents the function of a heart protector above and beyond the mechanics. It improves the heart's function when exercising by toning and strengthening the cardiac muscle. This characteristic demonstrates how hawthorn improves the heart's symphony of contractions and motions, which is consistent with the guide's primary theme.

Hawthorne's use in conventional European medicine as a remedy for congestive heart failure demonstrates its historical significance as a guardian of heart-health. The method of the guide, which combines ancient knowledge with current insight, is similar to this relationship between tradition and modern thinking.

Harmonizing with Drugs

The hawthorn's interaction with cardiac medicines is a fascinating chapter in the saga. Hawthorn may enhance the effectiveness of blood pressure medications when taken in conjunction with them. However, it is important to give serious thought to how prescription and herbal assistance work together. The guide promotes holistic dialogues with a doctor about using hawthorn while taking cardiac drugs, just as it does with holistic treatments.

A Flavorful Blessing

The benefits of hawthorn go beyond its medical value; it has a wonderfully sweet taste that enhances a variety of gourmet dishes. When homemade ketchup is infused with hawthorn essence, it transcends the role of a simple condiment to become a gastronomic declaration of heart-health. This incorporation of hawthorn's flavor into common dishes reflects the guide's topic, which explores herbal treatments as nutrition for the heart as well as cures.

The Hawthorn Ritual

As the end of summer approaches, a yearly tradition begins. The ripe and ready hawthorn berries beckon the herbalist's hands. A half-gallon tincture is created, a liquid elixir that reflects the guide's all-encompassing journey. The daily use of a tincture, a communion with the gifts of nature, echoes the relationship between hawthorn and heart-health. Hawthorn's designation as a "food" herb fits with the theme of the guide, which is a celebration of herbs as allies in nutrient and health-related endeavors.

As we wrap up this part, keep in mind that Hawthorn's protection of cardiovascular health is more than simply a feat of science; it is evidence of the symbiotic interaction between nature and our health. Hawthorn's tones reverberate in the complex symphony of heart-health, producing a tune that captures the essence of Exploring Herbal Approaches for heart-health.

3.2 Hawthorn Lifestyle Integration Techniques

Hawthorn appears as a colorful thread in the vast tapestry of heart-centered life, weaving its advantages into the fabric of daily activities. Beyond merely indulging, embracing Hawthorn's offers means integrating them into one's life in a way that supports the guide's overarching theme of heart-health.

- Add some hawthorn tincture to your everyday routine to make your days more enjoyable. Carefully crafted, this hawthorn essence liquid becomes a ritual of heart-nourishing purpose, smoothly integrating with the guide's holistic viewpoint.

- Brew some hawthorn tea and let the tastes and benefits permeate your periods of introspection and relaxation. Think about how this straightforward action fits into the symphony of heart-health you are developing as you sip.

- Embrace the sweet flavor of hawthorn in your culinary ventures, advises Culinary

Magic. Create special sauces with it, add it to ketchup, or experiment with sweets that have the flavor of heart-health in every mouthful.

- Create herbal blends by combining hawthorn with supplementary herbs to create heart-healthy mixes. These mixtures turn into a lovely way to interact with hawthorn's essence, whether it's an energizing morning infusion or a peaceful evening elixir.

- Hawthorn should be used as part of your mindfulness exercises. Its heart-guardian symbolism perfectly complements meditation and deepens your journey toward inner peace.

- Discover hawthorn-infused oils for relaxing massages or fragrant baths with Wellness-Infused Oils. The guide's strategy of tying heart-health to holistic experiences resonates with this tactile integration of hawthorn.

- Harvest hawthorn berries to connect with the seasonal cycles of nature. Gathering these gifts from the ground recalls the guide's exhortation to live in harmony with nature.

Keep in mind that each decision you make affects the harmony of your heart's well-being when you incorporate hawthorn into your way of life. A testament to the comprehensive relationship between nature's wisdom and the vibrancy of your heart, the hawthorn thread that was woven with care and devotion becomes a part of your story.

3.3 Culinary Adventures with Hawthorn: Enhancing Your Dishes

Hawthorn appears as a savory muse in the world of food, luring you on an alluring voyage of culinary discovery. Its presence goes beyond just being an ingredient; it presents a chance to flavor your recipes with the essence of heart-health, flawlessly integrating with the guide's all-encompassing perspective.

- Enhance your culinary creativity by including hawthorn in sauces, according to Dynamic Sauces. Hawthorn's sweet undertones complement both sweet and savory recipes, giving them depth and a dash of heart-warming flavor.

- Hawthorn should be a part of your daily routines for filling breakfasts. Hawthorn's sweet tones transform into a delicious ingredient that sets a heart-healthy tone for the day in anything from porridge to yogurt parfaits.

- Craft beverages that reflect the holistic wellness philosophy of the guide are called Vibrant Beverages. Hawthorn may be added to herbal teas, smoothies, and mocktails to make beverages that will not only satisfy your thirst but also be good for your heart.

- Engage in desert alchemy by incorporating hawthorn into your baked treats. Hawthorn's sweet personality enriches your delicacies with heart-nourishing appeal, whether they are cakes, muffins, or even homemade ice cream.

- With the help of relishes flavored with hawthorn, everyday foods may be transformed into outstanding masterpieces. A symphony of flavors that promotes heart-health is created when its flavor is combined with fruits and a hint of spice.

- Fusion food: Experiment with international flavors by adding hawthorn to a variety of dishes. Due to its adaptability, you can combine it with a variety of ingredients to produce fusion food that is both creative and healthy.

- Seasonal festivities: Let Hawthorn inspire your culinary festivities as the seasons shift. Put its essence into foods that symbolize the passing of time to give each celebration a touch of heart wellness.

Hawthorn's culinary explorations go beyond the sense of taste and transform into an emotional trip. In addition to enjoying the tastes of each meal, you are also creating a story about your overall health—a complex storyline in which the hawthorn flavors blend with the symphony of your heart's vigor.

3.4 Serving hawthorn with flair: presentation and enjoyment

Enhancing the heart-health experience includes the art of presentation and enjoyment in addition to the substance of the nutrients. Hawthorn serves as a blank canvas on which to create a culinary masterpiece that is consistent with the holistic philosophy of the guide thanks to its heart-nourishing qualities.

- Visual Delight: Add the vivacity of hawthorn to your display. Its deep crimson color creates a visually appealing flare for foods and drinks, creating the ideal environment for an amazing culinary experience.

- Hawthorn garnishes may elevate your dishes, according to Thoughtful Garnishes. These finishing touches, such as a dusting of dried hawthorn petals or a drizzle flavored with hawthorn, not only improve flavor but also show your dedication to heart-health.

- Artful Plating: Create artistic plates using hawthorn as the focal point.

Arrange meals with hawthorn-infused ingredients so that they reflect the harmonious fusion of tastes and the heart-healthy effects.

- Let each dish convey a tale through culinary storytelling. As you serve, discuss the significance of hawthorn to make a meaningful connection between your culinary creations and the study of herbal methods for heart-health.

- Heart-Healthy Atmosphere: Construct an environment that enhances the essence of hawthorn. Carefully set the table, possibly with hawthorn leaves or blooms, to beckon a holistic symphony that resonates with heart well-being.

- Consider each meal as a Mindful moment, according to the phrase. Let your focus dwell on the aromas, textures, and heart-nurturing purpose that each mouthful represents as you enjoy foods flavored with hawthorn.

- Share your hawthorn-infused creations with your loved ones to extend the bounty's benefits. The comprehensive idea of the guide is embodied in the act of sharing, which nurtures not only your own heart but also the hearts of others around you.

Hawthorn is a fruit that, when prepared creatively, goes beyond mere nutrition to become a multimodal celebration of heart-health. Each dish, garnish, and arrangement serves as a visual representation of the harmonious blend of tastes, colors, and overall design goals. You are not only treating your palate with each meal, but you are also absorbing the spirit of "Exploring Herbal Approaches for heart-health."

3.5 Perfect Moments: Selecting Hawthorn's Best Moments

Timing takes on the form of a delicate dance in the choreography of heart-health. Choosing the right times to invite hawthorn's presence increases its effect when it comes to enjoying its advantages. The comprehensive subject of the guide is fundamentally woven into the essence of hawthorn, bringing the rhythm of nature into our daily lives.

- Morning Awakening: Start your day with rituals filled with hawthorn. In keeping with the holistic tenet of the guide, a cup of hawthorn tea or a drop of medicine becomes a morning toast to heart wellness.

- Hawthorn can help you channel the lunchtime energy into your daily activities. Hawthorn delivers a noontime rejuvenation that resonates with the symphony of well-being, whether in your meals or as a cool beverage.

- Include hawthorn before meals to create a harmonious pre-meal environment. Its capacity to aid digestion ties in with the guide's emphasis on holistic well-being by establishing a rhythmic harmony between the body and the heart.

- Evening Reflection: As the day comes to an end, embrace hawthorn. The guide's emphasis on fostering the heart's symphony is in line with how its soothing qualities offer a gradual transition into times of introspection and rest.

- Incorporate mindfulness into your hawthorn consumption with Mindful Moments. Let your attention linger on the flavors, feelings, and goal of heart care with each sip or taste, matching the guide's all-encompassing approach.

- Let the seasons lead your hawthorn moments with Seasonal Serenade. By adjusting your hawthorn rituals to follow how nature evolves, you may establish a harmonious relationship with the planet's ever-evolving rhythms.

- Ritualistic Connection: Create a unique hawthorn ritual as a symbol of your dedication to heart-health. These rituals echo the guide's exhortation to integrate nature's blessings into our everyday lives, whether it is through a daily cup of tea or a seasonal tincture.

Keep in mind that when you choose the ideal times for hawthorn, each decision becomes a note in the symphony of heart wellness. Hawthorn's presence resonates with the spirit of the guide, whether it's the first light of morning or the peace of the evening, encouraging a holistic link between nature's knowledge and the rhythm of your heart.

3.6 Choosing Doses: Finding the Right Balance with Hawthorn

Hawthorn appears as a crucial thread that has to be carefully woven into the tapestry of a heart-centered existence. Finding the right dose balance involves more than simply adjusting the amount; it's a subtle dance that aligns with the guide's all-encompassing approach to heart care.

- The advantages of hawthorn blossom in moderation, much as a symphony finds its beauty in the harmony of sounds. Two cups of hawthorn tea per day is the general recommendation, echoing the holistic ethos of the guide and allowing nature's gift to work in harmony with your well-being.

- Recognize that every person's body and requirements are different by thinking of them as personal symphonies. The appropriate dose depends on some variables, including age, health, and individual reactions. To plan your hawthorn trip, pay attention to your body's signals and think about consulting a specialist.

- Dosage goes beyond quantitative measurements; it's a composition of hawthorn's inclusion in your comprehensive routine. Think about how hawthorn fits in with other heart-healthy routines to support the guide's central idea of linked well-being.

- Dialogues and Collaboration: When integrating hawthorn with drugs, have a dialogue with healthcare specialists. Just as musicians cooperate to produce harmonies and melodies. This conversation is in line with the guide's plea for an all-encompassing approach to heart-health.

- Create a ritual around your hawthorn dosage, such as sipping mindfully on a cup of tea or taking a daily droplet of tincture. These rituals transform from simple times of ingestion into symphonies of heart support, mirroring the guide's notion of the relationship between well-being and nature.

Hawthorne-style navigation is a nuanced skill, similar to leading a symphony. Remember that each sip or tincture becomes a note in the vast composition of heart-health as you adjust the balance. Your hawthorn journey reflects the entire core of "Exploring Herbal Approaches for heart-health," much like a well-played tune resonates in harmony.

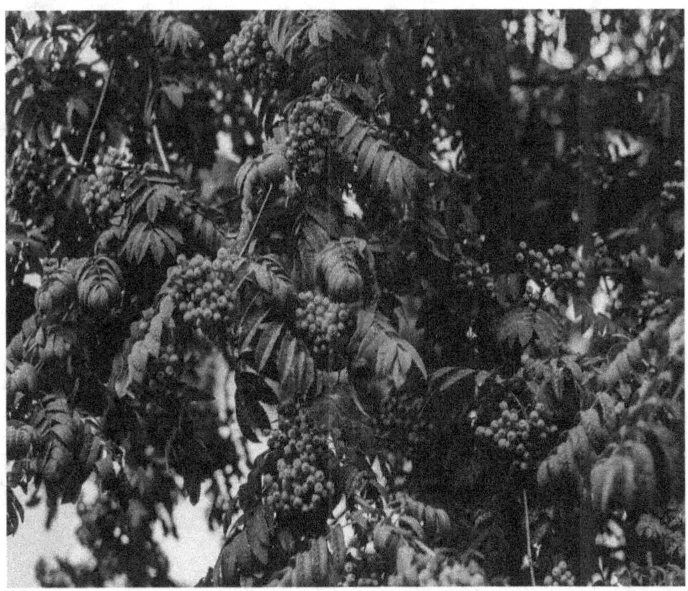

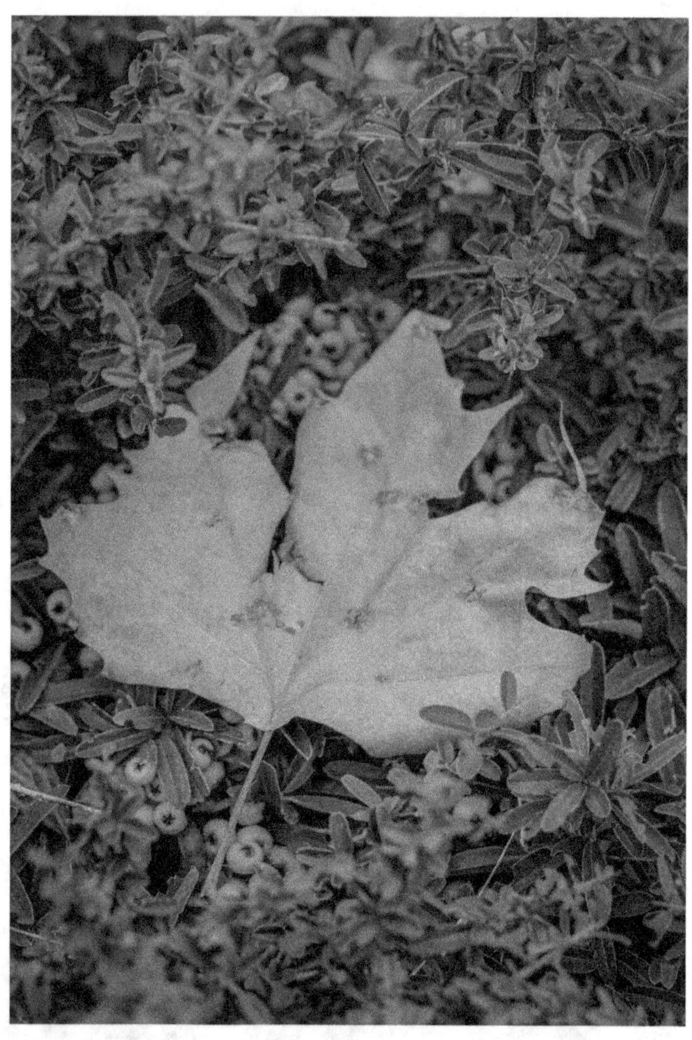

CHAPTER FOUR: Rooibos Tea: Calming Sips for Your Heart

4.1 The Heartfelt Effect of Rooibos on Cardiovascular Wellness

Rooibos Tea: Soothing Sips for Your Heart" after traveling through the serene landscape of heart-health. Here, in the middle of the health symphony, we investigate the gentle embrace of Rooibos, a tea that personifies coziness and tenderness. The overall essence of the guide and the essence of Rooibos combine in these pages to create a story of calming sips and heart-nourishing peace.

A Symphony of Flavor: The Elegance of Rooibos

In this chapter, the tea Rooibos, which is known for its heart-healthy properties as well as its exquisite flavor, emerges as a colorful character. The guide's topic of investigating herbal treatments for heart-health connects with the delicate dance of light, woody, and somewhat sweet sounds in it. The warmth and tint that result during roasting serve as a tangible example of Rooibos' attraction.

Quercetin's Blessing: Heartfelt Benefits of Rooibos

Rooibos tea has a host of heart-healthy advantages in addition to its endearing appeal. Rooibos has a significant amount of quercetin, which stands out as a cornerstone amid the variety of minerals and antioxidants. The ability of Rooibos to lower blood pressure, reduce inflammation, and influence cholesterol levels complements the holistic idea of the guide and puts it in tune with the symphony of heart wellness.

A Gentle Friend: Rooibos's Graceful Characteristics

The gentleness of Rooibos extends to its chemical make-up, which is devoid of oxalates and low in tannins. It is therefore a heart-healthy option, especially for people who are prone to kidney stones. The guide's exploration of herbal medicines that are in line with nature's wisdom reflects the symphony of Rooibos's qualities, which are created to nourish and care.

A Cup of Comfort: Rooibos's Ritual of Care

A cup of Rooibos is more than simply a drink; it's a ritual of solace and tenderness. Let its essence embrace you while you enjoy its tastes, bringing you moments of peace that are consistent with the entire investigation of the guide. Rooibos transforms into a symbol of self-care, a symphonic note in the tune of heart-health.

Therapeutic Symphony: Rooibos in Blends

Rooibos is used in medicinal mixes as a mellow component as well as for solitary use. Its gentle, calming nature serves as a link between Rooibos and other herbs, resulting in symphonies of healing that reflect the holistic viewpoint of the guide. These mixtures transform into elixirs of well-being that create harmony throughout the body.

A Toast to Wellness: The Generosity of Rooibos

You are invited to liberally enjoy Rooibos' advantages. Its accommodating nature allows for one or two cups each day, reflecting the guide's all-encompassing strategy for fostering heart-health via natural lifestyle choices. This request to partake in some Rooibos serves as a show of appreciation for the gift of good heart-health.

Holistic Symphony: Rooibos in Your Cup

Keep in mind that each drink of Rooibos contributes to the holistic symphony you are creating for the health of your heart. Within your cup, the harmony of tastes, the cocoon of comfort, and the essence of heart support may be felt. Rooibos is a representation of the guide's central premise, which is an exploration of herbal medicines that align with the liveliness of your heart.

As Rooibos' narrative comes to a close, it plays out like a tranquil song, a tribute to the harmony of heart-health. Its gentle embrace, which is tinged with tenderness and sustenance, mirrors the spirit of "Exploring Herbal Approaches for heart-health."

4.2 Sip by Sip: Approaches to Embrace Rooibos in Daily Life

Rooibos comes as a comforting brushstroke on the canvas of heart-centered life, coloring ordinary moments with its warm embrace. A symphony of heart wellness is created by integrating Rooibos into one's life in a way that resonates with the overall core of the guide, not merely by consuming it.

- Start your day peacefully with a cup of Rooibos tea—a nod to the guide's topic of promoting heart-health. Its mild, woody flavor serves as a calming undertone for the dawn's emergence.

- Midday Reprieve: Indulge in Rooibos at lunchtime. Its mildly sweet aromas provide a moment of calm, in keeping with the guide's advice to integrate heart care into your everyday routine.

- Evening Tranquility: Relax at the end of the day with Rooibos' soothing company. With the sun setting, Rooibos' warm color echoes the guide's theme of accepting heart support during reflective times.

- Create a daily routine around sipping Rooibos to appreciate its aromas and recognize its heart-nourishing properties. These drinks serve as evidence of the guide's all-encompassing wellness philosophy.

- Add Rooibos to your culinary masterpieces to achieve "Culinary Harmony." Its delicate flavor pairs wonderfully with a variety of foods, reflecting the guide's examination of herbal remedies as heart nutrition.

- Harmonious blends are made by combining Rooibos with other herbs that are good for the heart. The appeal for a complete symphony of well-being is echoed throughout the guide, and each cup becomes a sip of harmony.

- Approaching the use of Rooibos with awareness In keeping with the guide's idea of intentionally researching herbal remedies, let each drink be an act of presence.

Remember that each moment becomes a note in the magnificent composition of heart wellness as you enjoy Rooibos drink by sip. Rooibos's presence harmonizes with the guide's core themes, whether it's a morning wakeup, a noon break, or an evening reflection—unveiling the guide's "Exploring Herbal Approaches for heart-health Symphony.

4.3 Culinary Pairings: Rooibos' Delight Infused Meals

In the world of cooking, Rooibos reveals itself as a flexible ingredient, enhancing recipes with a special fusion of taste and coziness. The process of introducing Rooibos into your meals goes beyond merely indulging; it's a culinary adventure that aligns with the holistic philosophy of the guide and infuses heart-health into every morsel.

- Breakfast Elegance: Rooibos' delicate touch will elevate your morning meals. Utilize it in smoothie bowls, yogurt parfaits, or oatmeal to support the guide's recommendation to start the day with heart well-being.

- Craft soul-nourishing soups using Rooibos, according to Soulful Soups. Its warm, woodsy undertones blend with numerous ingredients to provide a symphony of tastes that mirror the guide's all-encompassing perspective.

- Culinary Elixirs: Try Rooibos-infused sauces and salads. Each drip transforms into a culinary elixir that honors both flavor and heart-health, much like the guide's examination of herbal remedies.

- Enticing Entrees: Rooibos will elevate your main courses." Use it to flavor braising liquids, glazes, and marinades to create a culinary experience that reflects the guide's emphasis on incorporating heart-health into daily life.

- Delectable Desserts:Transform sweets into delights that nourish the heart with The guide's guiding principle—exploring herbal remedies as joyous nourishment—resonates with the way that Rooibos' somewhat sweet undertones complement baked foods and sweet snacks.

- Herbal Harmonies: Blend Rooibos with other herbs that assist the heart. Create herbal concoctions that, in keeping with the holistic idea of the guide, enhance not only the flavor of your culinary creations but also their heart-nurturing qualities.

- Celebratory Feasts: Celebrate with Rooibos-infused meals. Let Rooibos be a part of your feasts, infusing each gathering with taste and heartfelt purposes, similar to the discovery of overall well-being in the guide.

Remember that each dish becomes a note in the culinary symphony of heart wellness as you infuse your meals with Rooibos' joy. The presence of Rooibos, like a culinary stroke, lends warmth and care to your meals, mirroring the core idea of "Exploring Herbal Approaches for Heart-Health."

4.4 Serving Rooibos: From Cozy Evenings to Energizing Mornings

The process of serving Rooibos goes beyond the simple preparation of a beverage and develops into a skillful presentation that corresponds with the entire idea of the guide. The presence of Rooibos harmonizes with daily cycles from dark to morning, creating a symphony of heart wellness.

- Evening Embrace: Serve Rooibos during the tranquil hours of the evening. It's comforting flavor and warm tint create a cocoon of coziness that echoes the guide's advice to tend to the heart during downtime.

- Morning Awakening Start your mornings with a cup of Rooibos, advises Morning Awakening. Its mild aromas serve as an invigorating beginning that mirrors the concept of the guide, which explores herbal methods to enliven the heart.

- Midday Revival. Add Rooibos to your lunchtime breaks to experience Whether it's a calming sip or a cool iced version, Rooibos becomes a friend that complements the guide's guiding principle of integrating daily routines and heart wellness.

- **Sharing with Loved Ones:** Serve Rooibos to loved ones as a token of your heartfelt concern for them. Rooibos's presence reflects the focus of the guide on sharing the journey of well-being, whether it be during gatherings or private times.

- **Ritualistic Cups:** Establish Rooibos serving customs. Make drinking each cup a focused moment that invites you to connect with the essence of heart wellness. This ritual will embody the guide's comprehensive inquiry.

- **Culinary Creations:** Serve culinary items that have been Rooibos-infused. Every dish, from sauces to desserts, is made more heart-nourishing by the use of Rooibos, reflecting the guide's examination of herbal cooking techniques.

- **Quiet Reflections:** Rooibos should be available for quiet reflections. In keeping with the guide's concept of accepting heart support in moments of awareness, let its tastes enhance your reflection.

Keep in mind that each cup of Rooibos becomes a note in the symphony of heart wellness as you serve it. Rooibos's presence harmonizes with the spirit of "Exploring Herbal Approaches for heart-health," creating a story that covers the whole range of everyday living, from calming evenings to energetic mornings.

4.5 Timing Your Teacup: The Best Times to Enjoy Rooibos's Benefits

The comprehensive approach to heart-health outlined in the guide is consistent with the thoughtful decision to savor Rooibos tea. Timing turns into a delicate art that embraces the essence of well-being while producing a rhythm that chimes with the everyday symphony.

- Dawn's Awakening: Invite Rooibos into your mornings The peaceful presence of Rooibos transforms into a calming ritual as the sun rises, complementing the guide's examination of herbal methods for energizing the heart.

- Midday Nourishment: Add Rooibos to your lunch. Its warmth provides a moment of solace and echoes the guide's theme of fusing daily routines with heart care.

- Sunset Serenity: Relax at the end of the day with Rooibos' company in The subtle sweetness of the sun's tones as it sets contributes to the peaceful atmosphere that the guide emphasizes is important for accepting heart support during reflective periods.

- **Pre-Meal Prelude:** Take Rooibos before meals. The guide's holistic philosophy and its capacity to promote digestion are in harmony, creating the ideal environment for nourishing the heart.

- Mindful Moments: Incorporate Rooibos into your moments. In keeping with the spirit of the guide, which is to explore herbal treatments with intention, while you drink, let your consciousness linger on the tastes and the goal of heart wellness.

- Communal Connections: Speak Rooibos to your family and friends. Rooibos's presence echoes the demand for heart-nourishing interactions made throughout the guide, whether in large gatherings or private chats.

- Restful Nights: Use Rooibos to relax at night. The guide's comprehensive concept of healing the heart during moments of repose is in line with how its relaxing qualities create a peaceful transition into periods of rest.

Timing your tea cup turns it into a well-being orchestration—a deliberate dance that harmonizes with your heart's symphony. Every time you choose to drink Rooibos, you are adding a note to the great composition of heart-health and resonating the spirit of "Exploring Herbal Approaches for Heart-Health" with each sip.

4.6 Dosage Insights: Measuring Rooibos' Tranquil Influence

Beyond taste, navigating the Rooibos world requires a careful balance that is consistent with the guide's all-encompassing approach to heart-health. Finding the ideal dosage turns into an investigation of harmony, where the calming effects of Rooibos interact with your well-being.

- **Gentle Moderation:** The advantages of Rooibos emerge in moderation, much as a symphony finds its beauty in the proper harmony of notes. The guide's holistic approach to fostering the well-being of the heart is in line with drinking two to three cups each day.

- **Personal Symphony:** Be aware that every person's body reacts uniquely. The appropriate dose depends on some variables, including age, health, and personal resonance. Pay attention to your body's signals while thinking about getting professional advice.

- **Holistic Integration:** Dosage isn't just a number; it's Rooibos's presence in your daily activities as a harmonious whole. Put it into circumstances that reflect the guideline of incorporating heart fitness into all facets of life.

- Conversations and Harmony: Converse with healthcare specialists when combining Rooibos with drugs, much as musicians cooperate to create harmonic tunes. This conversation is in line with the guide's comprehensive examination of cardiac support.

- Ritualistic Wisdom: Create a Rooibos ritual by taking a moment each day to appreciate its tastes and acknowledge its heart-nourishing qualities, according to ritualistic wisdom. These practices continue the guide's subject of attentive participation in the path to well-being.

Remember that each cup contributes a note to the symphony of heart wellness as you gauge Rooibos' calming effect. Every sip brings the spirit of harmony, mirroring your efforts to create peaceful moments through "Exploring Herbal Approaches for Heart-Health."

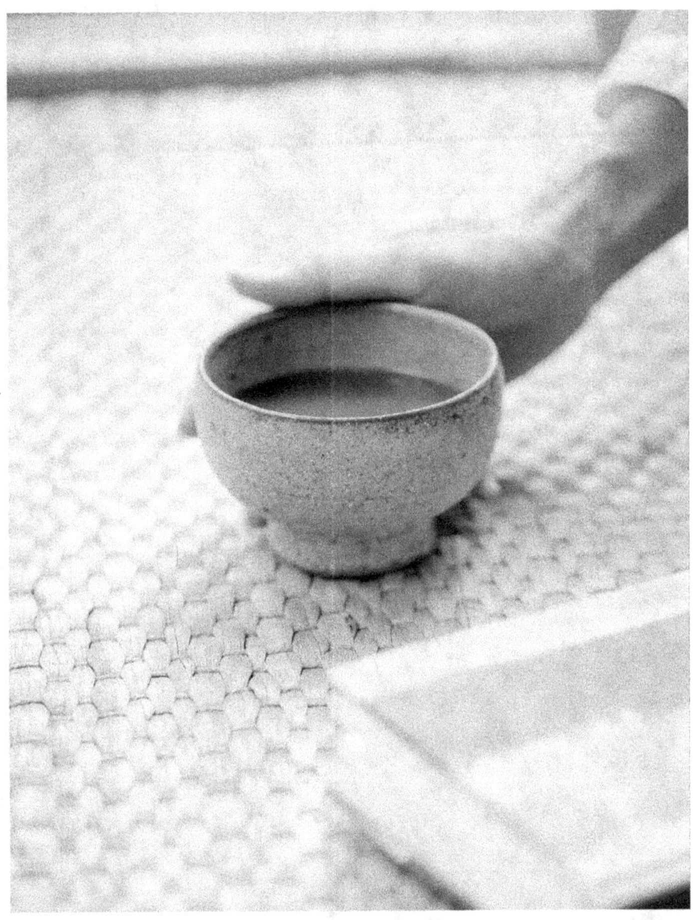

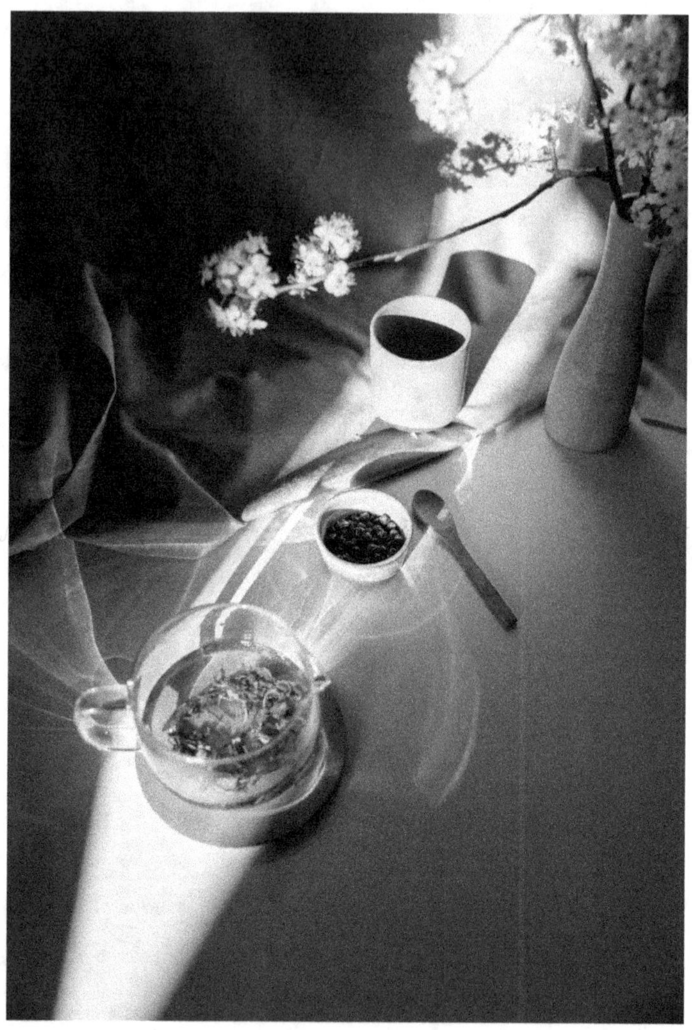

CHAPTER FIVE: Motherwort: Embrace the Heart's Calm

5.1 Motherwort's Gentle Touch on Heart Health"

This chapter, Motherwort: Embrace the Heart's Calm," is in line with the overall theme of the guide, which is to explore herbal remedies for heart health. Motherwort takes center stage in the symphony of heart-supporting herbs, giving its distinctive song of peace and healing.

The Alchemy of Motherwort

Discover motherwort, an herb that provides comforting and well-balanced advice. The product is a very good option for men and women looking for tonic cardiovascular health because of its nature, which is implied by its name alone. Motherwort's essence ties nicely with the book's emphasis on heart health.

Leonurine's Heartfelt Symphony

The heart-supporting qualities of motherwort are evidence of its makeup. A vital ingredient in Motherwort, leonurine, performs the function of a vasodilator, or conductor of open channels for optimal blood flow. This fits in perfectly with the guide's examination of herbs that promote the healthy operation of the heart.

Nurturing the Nervous Symphony

Motherwort has effects that go beyond cardiovascular health; it also has nervine properties. Its capacity to soothe anxiety by calming and toning the nervous system is consistent with the guide's holistic idea of uniting the heart and head. Motherwort provides a gentle hug for the health of the heart as it tends to the nervous system.

The Elegance of Tinctures

The narrative of Motherwort is not complete without the shape that was chosen. The heart-supporting alkaloids in motherwort are transported through tinctures, which use alcohol as the solvent. This story of herbal knowledge ties in with the guide's topic of discovering herbal remedies in a way that brings out the best in each plant.

A Tradition of Heart Care

Motherwort is known for its history as a traditional cardiotonic herb and as a protector against heart palpitations and arrhythmias. This history is evidence of its efficacy and fits well with the guide's investigation of herbs that are compatible with the beat of the heart. The very scientific name of Motherwort, which contributes a note to the symphony of heart support, echoes this heritage.

Resonance and Contraindications

Keep in mind that Motherwort's resonance encompasses both advantages and considerations as you immerse yourself in its warm embrace. The guide's focus on informed well-being finds its echo here, offering its calming influence. **Pregnant or breastfeeding women** should exercise caution, which is in line with the guide's advice to approach herbal wellness with awareness and information.

Harmonizing with Expert Advice

The story of Motherwort serves as a helpful reminder of the value of expert advice when it comes to heart health. The guide promotes comprehensive exploration while simultaneously stressing the need to make well-informed choices. The guide's concept of an informed journey is echoed in Motherwort's melody, which develops into a harmonic interplay of knowledge and tenderness.

Motherwort's role as a soft refrain in the symphony of heart support is evidence of the herb's capacity to calm, heal, and harmonize. The everlasting song of well-being is woven into its essence, just like it is in "Exploring Herbal Approaches for Heart-Health," with care and intention.

5.2 Accepting the Presence of Motherwort in Your Regimen

Motherwort serves as a compassionate companion during the heart-centered journey and lends its calming influence to your wellness routine. Adopting Motherwort is more than just a decision; it's a deliberate action that reflects the comprehensive philosophy of the guide and integrates heart-health into your everyday activities.

- Integrating with Intention: When incorporating Motherwort into your routine, be sure to do it with intention. Let it embody the idea of the guide, which emphasizes embracing heart wellness while maintaining mindfulness and purpose.

- Daily Rituals: Create regular routines to recognize the soothing effects of motherwort. Let Motherwort be a part of your heart-centered rituals, whether it be a little time of solitude or a committed stop.

- Nurturing the Heart-Mind: Motherwort's capacity to soothe the nervous system serves as a link between the heart and the mind in the phrase "Nurturing the Heart-Mind." Allow its effect to foster this interaction as you incorporate it into your routine, in keeping with the guide's examination of holistic well-being.

- Tincture Wisdom: When using motherwort, use the form that best accentuates its qualities, advises Tincture Wisdom. The subject of the guide is to explore herbal remedies that are in tune with the requirements of the heart. Tinctures, with their capacity to retain and unleash their benefits, match this idea.

- Professional Conversations: As you incorporate Motherwort into your routine, have discussions with healthcare experts. This conversation supports the idea of holistic treatment and mirrors the guide's focus on informed well-being.

- **Mindful Adjustments:** Observe how Motherwort's presence affects your well-being by making mindful adjustments. Pay attention to your body's signals and modify as necessary, echoing the guide's appeal for attentive participation on the road toward heart-health.

- **Heartful Expressions:** Express your relationship with Motherwort by writing in a diary or other forms of artistic expression. This kind of introspection is consistent with the guide's discussion of cardiac support as a comprehensive and individual journey.

As you welcome Motherwort into your routine, keep in mind that every decision you make contributes to the harmony of your heart's health. Motherwort's affect connects with the essence of "Exploring Herbal Approaches for Heart-Health," generating a story that harmonizes with your holistic journey, whether it be through a tincture, a ritual, or a chat with a professional.

5.3 Culinary Alchemy: Incorporating Motherwort into Your Cuisine

Motherwort is a novel addition to the world of culinary experimentation and an alchemical contribution that fits with the holistic spirit of the guide. It's not just about adding taste when you include Motherwort in your cooking; it's a symphony that integrates heart wellness into the craft of nourishing.

- Flavorful Infusions: Try infusing the mild essence of motherwort into your meals. Let it blend in with other ingredients in sauces, soups, and other dishes, mirroring the guide's examination of herbal techniques as culinary allies.

- Heartfelt Elixirs: Create heartfelt elixirs in the kitchen by adding motherwort to marinades and sauces. Each drop transforms into a heart-nourishing note that resonates with the guide's topic of investigating herbal methods for heart-health.

- Savory Symphonies: Incorporate Motherwort into savory dishes to give your meals a relaxing effect. This harmony echoes the guide's advice to include heart support in daily life's rhythm.

- **Sweet Offerings:** Infuse Motherwort's fragrance into desserts to let its calming effect reverberate with sweet delights. The investigation of heart wellness as a holistic journey throughout the guide is consistent with this fusion.

- **Mindful Creations:** Create attentively when you include motherwort in your dishes. Let each contribution reflect the guide's theme of intentionally accepting heart support by making a conscious decision.

- **Culinary Conversations:** Share your culinary masterpieces with Motherwort to start discussions about heart-health and general well-being. This interaction is consistent with the guide's core message of strengthening bonds through caring from the heart.

- **Personal Explorations:** Accept motherwort-infused food as a part of your explorations. The guide's subject of embracing herbal treatments as a symphony of nourishment aligns with the idea that each plate becomes a canvas for your investigation of heart wellness.

As you use Motherwort in your cooking, keep in mind that each meal contributes a note to the gastronomic symphony of heart-health. Motherwort's presence harmonizes with the core of "Exploring Herbal Approaches for Heart-Health," just like herbs do in a recipe, to create a story that embraces taste and tenderness.

5.4 Presenting Comfort: Carefully Serving Motherwort

Motherwort assumes a role beyond nutrition in the presentational sphere; it becomes an offering of consolation and tenderness. Serving Motherwort is more than just setting a cup down; it's a sentimental act that fits with the overall idea of the guide and integrates heart wellness into meals.

- Gentle Beginnings: Start your day gently with Motherwort. Its morning appearance is consistent with the guide's examination of herbal methods for reviving the heart's rhythm.

- Heartfelt Midday Pause: Add Motherwort's calming touch to your midday break. In keeping with the guide's guiding principle of integrating heart wellness with daily activities, let it be a time of heartfelt respite.

- Tranquil Evenings: Enjoy a cup of motherwort as you wind down your nights in Its soothing qualities fit with the guide's focus on accepting heart assistance during reflective times.

- Ritualistic Moments: Create rituals centered on providing for Motherwort. Let each serving be a conscious note in the symphony of heart well-being, whether it's a certain period or a particular cup.

- Shared Connections: Serve Motherwort to loved ones to forge ties that are carefully woven. The examination of heart support as a journey shared with others around you in the guide connects with this deed.

- Presentation with Mindfulness: Serve Motherwort with Mindfulness. Be mindful of the cup, the environment, and the aim. This reinforces the guide's message that herbal remedies should be used mindfully.

- Heart-Centered Offerings: Infuse each serving of Motherwort with heart-centered intentions. Let your acts of kindness complement the guide's core message, which is to protect the health-heart.

Remember that each cup becomes a note in the symphony of heart wellness as you present Motherwort with care. Serving shows your commitment to providing comprehensive care in addition to providing sustenance. The inclusion of motherwort complements the theme of "Exploring Herbal Approaches for Heart-Health," forming a story that values both sustenance and comfort.

5.5 Time for Tranquility: Selecting Motherwort Moments

The option of when to appreciate Motherwort becomes a thoughtful one within the tempo of daily life, in keeping with the holistic theme of the guide. It's not simply a matter of timing when to welcome Motherwort's presence; it's also a matter of incorporating heart-health into your daily routine.

- Morning Serenity: Start your mornings with a cup of motherwort,.Let its relaxing influence usher in a peaceful day ahead, complementing the guide's investigation of herbal methods for energizing the heart.

- Midday Harmony: Fill your lunch break with the peace of Motherwort. Its presence provides a tender pause, in keeping with the guide's core message of integrating heart support into daily activities.

- Evening Reflection: Let Motherwort's embrace help you wind down your nights. Its soothing qualities fit with the guide's focus on heart support during reflective times

- Mindful Contemplation: Select peaceful periods for Motherwort to practice mindful meditation. The investigation of comprehensive well-being throughout the guide is resonant with its presence, whether it is during meditation or a brief period of silence.

- Shared Moments: Share Motherwort with close friends and family to create peaceful times. The guide's guiding principle of fostering heart connections via shared experiences is reflected in this deed.

- Moments of Self-Care: Include Motherwort in your regimen of self-care. Whether it's when reading, journaling, or taking a bath, let its presence complement the overall philosophy of the guide.

- Before Sleep: Consider capping up your day with a cup of Motherwort. As the guide explores heart support during repose, its relaxing effect serves as a gateway to pleasant evenings.

Remember that when you select the appropriate times for Motherwort, each decision adds a note to the harmony of your heart's health. Motherwort's presence fits with the spirit of "Exploring Herbal Approaches for Heart-Health," creating a story that connects with serenity and intention, whether it's a morning routine or a shared moment.

5.6 Balancing Acts: Establishing the Proper Motherwort Dosage"

Finding the proper dose of Motherwort within the tapestry of heart support becomes an inquiry of balance, mirroring the comprehensive view of well-being in the guide. The process of determining the right dose fits with the guide's core message of thoughtful and informed research.

- Gentle Beginnings: When adding motherwort to your regimen, start with a moderate dosage. Following the guide's premise of starting the herbal journey with awareness, follow your body's response.

- Personalized Harmony: Recognize that every person's body reacts differently. The best dose depends on some variables, including age, health, and resonance. Pay attention to your body's signals while thinking about getting professional advice.

- Incremental Adjustments: As you observe the results, gradually increase the dosage. This is consistent with the guide's emphasis on taking a holistic approach and giving your body time to establish its equilibrium.

- Professional Conversations: As you determine Motherwort's dose, have discussions with healthcare specialists. This conversation supports the guide's advice to make educated choices in the interest of maintaining heart-health.

- Mindful Observations: Observe the effects that various doses have on your well-being. In keeping with the guide's concept of attentive participation in the discovery of herbal treatments, pay attention to your body's reactions.

- Holistic integration: Consider including the dose in your holistic routine. Let it blend in with other care components, mirroring the guide's discussion of heart support as a symphony of well-being.

- Self-Care Ritual: As you determine the right dose, incorporate it into your self-care routine. Each dosage transforms into a deliberate act of love that resonates with the guide's all-encompassing strategy for nourishing the heart.

Remember that each decision you make contributes to the symphony of your heart's health as you negotiate the delicate balancing act of Motherwort's dose. The right amount of Motherwort harmonizes with the spirit of "Exploring Herbal Approaches for Heart-Health," creating a story that celebrates both balance and informed well-being, just as herbs combine harmoniously.

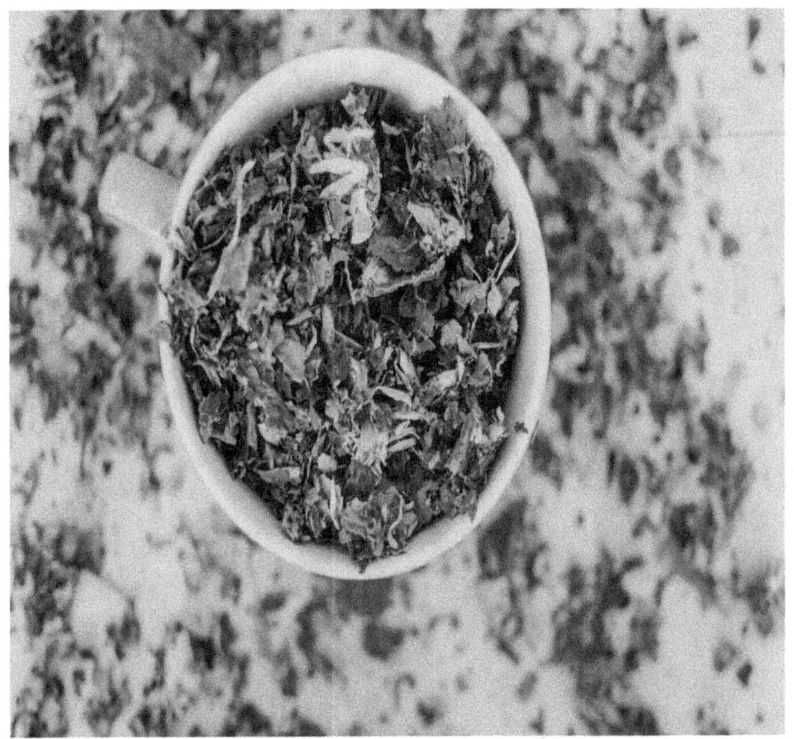

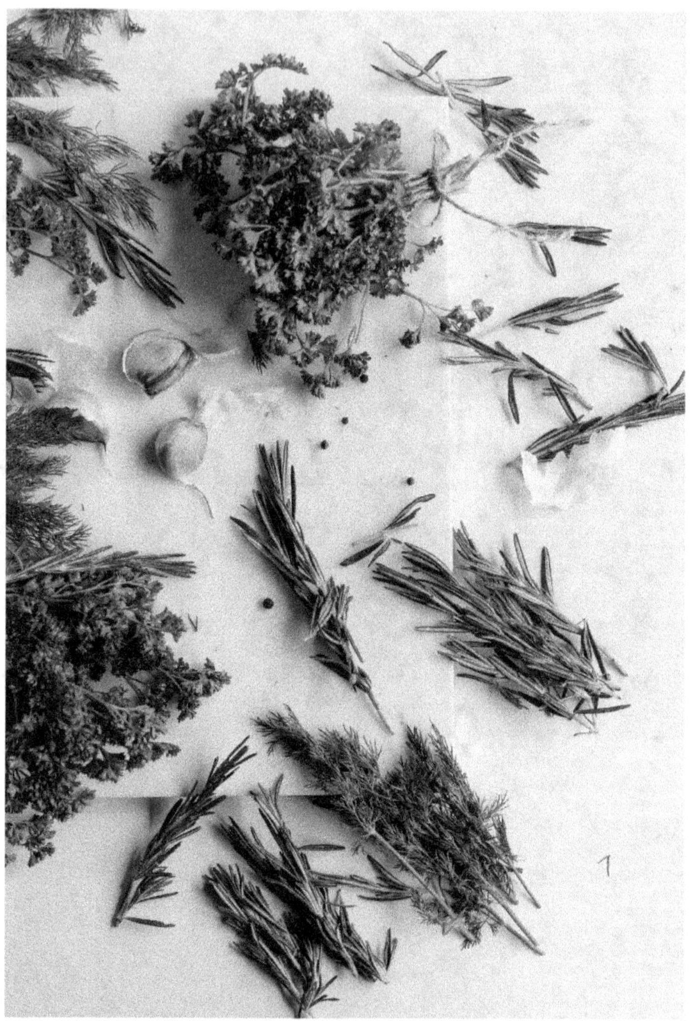

CHAPTER SIX: Ginger: A Spicy heart-health Support

6.1 Ginger: Zestful heart-health Support

Welcome to "Chapter 6: Ginger: Zestful heart-health Support," a chapter that relates to the main idea of the guide, which is to examine herbal methods for promoting heart-health. Among the wide variety of herbs that assist the heart, ginger stands out as a lively ally, adding its distinct flavor to the symphony of heart-health.

Ginger's Dynamic Healing

Ginger is a vibrant thread in the heart-healthy tapestry and a living example of how effective nature is at mending. Its capacity to reduce inflammation aligns with the guide's central tenet of holistic therapy, which takes the entire body into account.

Balancing Inflammation: Natural NSAIDs (anti-inflammatory drugs)

The effects of ginger on inflammation extend beyond the pages of the guide and become an important factor in cardiovascular health. Its ingredients, which are similar to those in NSAIDs, interact with the body's systems naturally, generating a harmony that mirrors the guide's comprehensive investigation.

Scientific Echoes of Healing

Studies conducted in the field of science indicate the heart-supporting properties of ginger. These parallels emphasize its significance and are consistent with the guide's focus on informed well-being. The research supporting ginger's effect on lipid and cholesterol levels supports the significance that ginger plays in heart-health.

Ginger's Heartfelt

Ginger plays a crucial role in the guide's culinary approach to heart fitness as a culinary herb. Its use in food and treatment chimes with the holistic idea, tying the act of nourishing into the path to wellness.

Culinary Symphony: From Slice to Sip

The guide recommends a straightforward but effective technique—using the genuine Ginger plant—to harness Ginger's heart-supporting effects. The act of slicing an inch-long piece and steeping it in tea fits with the guide's premise of using organic and conscientious methods. Ginger is infused into daily activities to mimic the beat of the heart.

Infusions of Wellness

With the addition of Ginger to the symphony of heart-supporting herbs, an innovative infusion comes to life. The herbs stated previously generate a mix when a slice is added, which is consistent with the guide's examination of herb pairings. Each drink creates a melodic note that promotes heart-health.

Rooted in Freshness and Potency

The story of Ginger's use goes beyond practicality; it's about appreciating nature's most recent gifts. The focus on the real plant in the novel is consistent with Ginger's strength. By becoming a decision that reflects the guide's ideals, the decision to utilize the fresh root becomes an embodiment of the comprehensive philosophy of the guide.

Ginger's Role in the Heart's Melody

The story of Ginger develops like a vivacious melody—a healing symphony of tastes. Ginger's vivid touch becomes a note that harmonizes with the heart's well-being, asking you to embrace its zing on the path of holistic health. Every element, from its influence on inflammation to its culinary presence, resonates with the essence of "Exploring Herbal Approaches for Heart-Health."

6.2 Creative Paths to Infuse Ginger into Your Routine

On the heart-supporting journey, adding ginger takes on a creative dimension, infusing your daily activities with its fiery flavor. The chapter "Creative Paths to Infuse Ginger into Your Routine" complements the guide's examination of herbal remedies by providing a variety of ways to embrace Ginger's vitality.

- Culinary Innovations: Add the distinct flavor of ginger to your recipes. Let its zesty flavor permeate your culinary creations, from soups to stir-fries, to reflect the guide's gastronomic examination of heart wellness.

- Nourishing Elixirs: Create elixirs that combine the heart-supporting properties of various herbs with the intensity of ginger. This innovative fusion weaves Ginger's touch into medicinal mixtures, echoing the guide's topic of herbal combinations.

- Morning Enlivenment: Start your day with a cup of ginger tea to get your day going. Its energizing nature fits with the guide's outlook on heart-health, which embraces the morning as a new day.

- Sip of Wellness: Make a revitalizing infusion by steeping ginger slices in water with a little vinegar. This intentional practice of drinking water fits with the guide's all-encompassing strategy for nurturing the heart.

- Dynamic Pairings: Blend ginger with other substances that help the heart. Let each combination be a movement in the heart-wellness symphony, mirroring the overall subject of the guide.

- Flavorsome Enhancements: Increase your water consumption by adding ginger slices, according to Flavorsome Enhancements. This straightforward action enhances hydration with a flavorful kick, in keeping with the guide's emphasis on making thoughtful decisions.

- Herbal Symphony: Blend ginger slices and the heart-healthy plants described before to create an herbal symphony. This innovative combination complements the guide's investigation of how to combine herbs for a holistic heart symphony.

As you incorporate Ginger into your daily routine, keep in mind that each creative avenue contributes a note to the harmony of your heart's health. The addition of ginger to your regimen resonates with the essence of "Exploring Herbal Approaches for Heart-Health," generating a narrative that honors both invention and care, just as herbs combine to make harmonious combinations.

6.3 Culinary Explorations: Adding Spice with Ginger

Ginger stands out as an alluring spice in the culinary world, supporting the guide's all-encompassing subject of embracing heart wellness via nutrition. The guide "Culinary Explorations: Adding Spice with Ginger" invites you to go on a savory adventure that echoes with the vigor of the heart.

- Flavorful Infusions: Add the zesty flavor of ginger to your culinary masterpieces. Let its zestful touch improve your meals, matching the guide's culinary examination of heart wellness, whether it is a dash in a sauce or a sprinkle in a marinade.

- Spice of Heart: Accept the power of ginger as a spice that not only titillates the palate but also warms the heart. This is consistent with the guide's premise of incorporating heart support into daily living.

- Culinary Harmony: Combine Ginger with other ingredients to make a delicious symphony. Let the mutual demands of the heart be echoed in each coupling, following the guide's idea of comprehensive discovery.

- Aromatic Delights: Enjoy the scent of ginger as it permeates your. The guide's The road emphasis on using the senses on the road toward wellness is consistent with the fragrance of the object.

- Nourishing Creations: Create foods that honor wellness and taste. Cooking with ginger becomes a culinary gesture that supports the guide's investigation of holistic nutrient intake.

- Mindful Additions: Be attentive while including ginger in your meals. Let each sprinkling be a deliberate act of tenderness, evoking the guide's emphasis on purposeful heart-nurturing.

- Fusion of Flavors: To make delectable mixtures, combine ginger with the previously stated herbs and substances. This combination relates to the guide's investigation of herbal mixtures that promote cardiac health.

Keep in mind that each addition becomes a note in the symphony of your heart's well-being as you and Ginger explore the world of food. The addition of ginger to your foods connects with the essence of "Exploring Herbal Approaches for Heart-Health," generating a narrative that embraces both flavor and sustenance. Herbs combine to produce harmonious flavors.

6.4 Serving Spice: The Versatility of Ginger in Culinary Delights"

Ginger's flexibility shines in the realm of culinary creation, reflecting the guide's all-encompassing strategy for promoting heart-health. The guide "Serving Spice: Ginger's Versatility in Culinary Delights" discusses the various ways that ginger enhances culinary delights while also striking a chord with the vigor of the heart.

- Culinary Showcases: Allow Ginger to take center stage in your recipes. Its presence shines a spotlight on tastes that are good for the heart, matching the guide's examination of well-being via food.

- Heartfelt Enhancements: Recognize ginger's function as an ally who supports the heart rather than merely a spice. This insight is consistent with the guide's core message of embracing all aspects of life for heart wellness.

- Culinary Artistry: Try out Ginger's various applications in your culinary masterpieces. The notion of comprehensive discovery is echoed throughout the guide with each addition, which acts as a brushstroke on the culinary canvas.

- Savor the Experience: Take pleasure in the tastes that Ginger incorporated into your food. Let the emphasis on thoughtful nutrition that improves heart-health permeate every mouthful, as it does throughout the guide.

- Heart-Centered Combinations: Blend ginger with a variety of ingredients to create flavorful combinations that are heart-centered. Each combination reflects the guide's investigation of all-encompassing care for the health of the heart.

- Present with Passion: When serving meals that have been seasoned with ginger, present them with passion. Let each dish represent your dedication to promoting heart-health, in keeping with the principles of the guide.

- Fusion of Taste: Combine Ginger with the heart-healthy herbs and spices listed above. The guide's research of blending ingredients for a comprehensive heart song connects with this fusion of tastes.

You should keep in mind that each meal you prepare becomes a note in the symphony of your heart's well-being as you embrace Ginger's variety in your culinary undertakings. The addition of ginger to your culinary creations connects with the concept of "Exploring Herbal Approaches for Heart-Health," generating a narrative that celebrates both flavor and culinary care. Herbs combine to produce harmonious flavors.

6.5 Timing the Spice: How and When to Benefit from Ginger"

With the guide's all-encompassing approach to heart fitness, the time of relishing Ginger's advantages assumes relevance. By picking the proper times to include Ginger into your day, "Timing the Spice: When to Enjoy Ginger's Benefits" inspires you to enjoy the rhythm of well-being.

- **Morning Awakening:** Start your day with drinks flavored with ginger in the morning. Ginger's energizing touch fits with the guide's concept of viewing the morning as a brand-new opportunity for heart-health.

- **Midday Vitality:** Add ginger's zingy taste to your midday meals. Let it speak to your heart's energy, reflecting the guide's emphasis on promoting well-being all day long.

- **Evening Comfort:** Relax in the evenings with a meal flavored with ginger. The guide's emphasis on heart support during periods of rest is echoed by the fragrance's calming but delicious scent.

- **Mindful Moments:** Select indulgent moments for Ginger while remaining aware. Allow Ginger's presence to complement the guide's examination of total participation, whether it is during meditation or a peaceful moment.

- **Shared Delights:** Share foods with loved ones that are flavored with ginger. Let your shared enjoyment reflect the guide's emphasis on strengthening relationships via common experiences.

- **Heartful Hydration:** Throughout the day, add ginger slices to your water for hearty hydration. This heart-healthy hydration is consistent with the guide's emphasis on deliberate decisions.

- Harmonious Combinations: When necessary, pair ginger with other heart-supporting ingredients. Each coupling should serve as a note in the symphony of heart-health, mirroring the overall subject of the guide.

As you welcome Ginger's advantages at this time, keep in mind that each decision you make adds a note to the harmony of your heart's health. The integration of Ginger's timing into your day connects with the concept of "Exploring Herbal Approaches for Heart-Health," generating a story that embraces both intention and energy, just as herbs mingle to produce harmonious tastes.

6.6 Dosage Decisions: Evaluating the Effect of Ginger on Your Health

An important choice in your heart-supporting path is how much ginger to take, which is in line with the guide's holistic approach to well-informed wellbeing. You are urged to walk this path mindfully by Dosage Decisions: Gauging Ginger's Impact on Your Well-Being, just as you would by the herbal remedies covered in the guide.

- Gradual Initiation: Start using ginger in a moderate amount. The guide emphasizes the importance of beginning the trip with conscious care; let your body's reaction serve as your guidance.

- Personalized Exploration: Be aware of the particular requirements of your body. Your optimum dose depends on some factors, including age and health. This individualized strategy fits with the guide's all-encompassing investigation.

- Incremental Modifications: As you evaluate Ginger's effects, progressively modify the dosage. This approach matches the premise of the guide, which is a comprehensive journey, by giving your body time to establish its balance.

- Professional communication: Have discussions with medical experts to decide on Ginger's dose in the best possible way. This conversation is in line with the guide's advice to make educated decisions in the quest for heart-health.

- Mindful Observations: Be mindful of the effects that various doses have on your well-being. In keeping with the guide's concept of attentive participation in the discovery of herbal treatments, pay attention to your body's reactions.

- Integral Wellness: Include Ginger's dose in your routine for whole wellness. Let it blend in with other care components, mirroring the guide's discussion of heart support as a symphony of well-being.

- Informed Choices: Before choosing Ginger's dose, make informed decisions by giving research and self-awareness priority. This parallels the guide's emphasis on making informed decisions by using all available information.

Keep in mind that each step you take to adjust the dosage of Ginger adds a note to the harmony of your heart's health. The dose of Ginger matches with the concept of "Exploring Herbal Approaches for Heart-Health," generating a story that praises both educated decisions and vitality, just as herbs combine to make harmonious combinations.

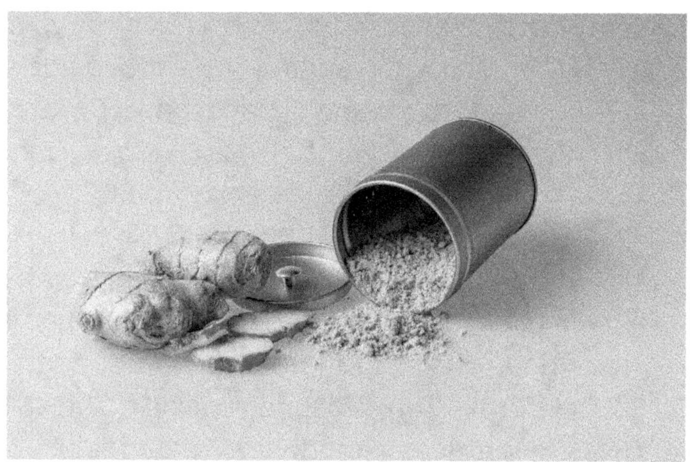

CHAPTER SEVEN: Cayenne Pepper: Igniting Heart Health

7.1 Cayenne Pepper's Fiery Boost to Cardiovascular Wellness

Cayenne Pepper: Igniting heart-health, a guide that explores herbal methods for nourishing the heart, resounds with the lively notes of the spice in the symphony of heart wellness. The title of the guide, Cayenne Pepper's Fiery Boost to Cardiovascular Wellness, ignites the fires of cardiovascular vigor.

Cayenne Pepper's Vigorous Resonance

Cayenne Pepper is a strong component on the path to heart-health and a symbol of the ferocious power of nature. The central concept of the guide, comprehensive heart care, resonates with the herb's reputation for promoting circulatory function.

Purification and Circulation: A Dynamic Dance

The detoxifying properties of cayenne pepper create a vivacious dance with blood cleansing. Its impact on blood flow fits in perfectly with the holistic idea of the guide, which embraces natural ingredients for heart-health.

Strengthening and Toning: Dilating Arteries

Cayenne's special ability to widen blood vessels serves as a reflection of the guide's topic of fostering heart strength. Its potential as a daily tonic is in line with the guide's appeal for comprehensive assistance that both sustains and energizes.

Cholesterol Control: A Flavorful Ally

The understanding of Cayenne's function in lowering cholesterol is consistent with the guide's use of herbs to promote general heart-health. Its presence turns into a tasty companion on the path to heart fitness.

The Blaze of Circulatory Power

The guide's topic of lively involvement with heart-health connects with the fiery effect that cayenne pepper has on the circulatory system. Cayenne is given heroic status by the audacious claim that it may prevent heart attacks, matching the guide's examination of the exceptional possibilities of plants.

Emergency Preparedness: A Tincture's Vigilance.

The guide's emphasis on preparation is in line with the preparedness of a Cayenne Pepper tincture. As the guide explores unusual remedies, the idea of Cayenne as an emergency clotting agent becomes a testament to the herb's skill.

Daily Incorporation: From Spicy to Sip

The prevalence of cayenne pepper in daily activities reflects the guide's recommendation to incorporate heart-supporting herbs into everyday activities. The incorporation of Cayenne into daily routines, whether it be by cooking with the powder or blending it into tea blends, connects with the examination of the holistic throughout the guide.

Rosy Chocolate Chai Tea: A delightful fusion

The Rosy Chocolate Chai Tea recipe's use of cayenne creates a savory representation of the guide's culinary journey. This mouthwatering concoction invites readers to appreciate heart support with every sip and reflects the topic of the guide, which is the mixing of taste and well-being.

The Emergency Potential of Cayenne: A Story of Clotting

This chapter's investigation of Cayenne Pepper's potential as an emergency clotting agent develops into a compelling story. With its ability to help people through difficult times, it supports the guide's message of holistic empowerment and encourages readers to explore further into the world of herbs.

Remember that each experience you have while you research the effects of cayenne pepper on heart-health becomes a note in the symphony of your heart's health. Cayenne Pepper's involvement in your heart-supporting journey connects with the concept of "Exploring Herbal Approaches for Heart-Health," generating a story that embraces both brightness and vigor, just as herbs combine to produce harmonious tastes.

7.2 Adding the Zest of Cayenne Pepper to Your Daily Life

A reflection of the guide's all-encompassing approach to heart fitness, Cayenne Pepper's vibrancy arises within the fabric of daily activities. This section, "Incorporating Cayenne Pepper's Zest into Your Daily Life," asks you to intentionally include the spicy flavor of cayenne throughout your day, mirroring the fundamental tenet of the guide.

- Culinary Infusion: Add the spiciness of cayenne to your culinary masterpieces. Let its vivid flavor permeate your meals as you explore the culinary discovery of heart wellness in the guide.

- Daily Tonic: Incorporate cayenne into your daily tonic to enliven your routine. This parallels the guide's theme of incorporating heart-healthy herbs into daily living.

- Spiced Beverages: Cayenne may be added to teas or other beverages to give them an energizing flavor. Let every drink, in keeping with the guide's all-encompassing participation, be a moment of heart-supporting energy.

- Dynamic Pairings: Combine cayenne with other substances that are good for the heart. Let the concept of the guide's harmonic integration for well-being be reflected in each combination.

- Morning Awakening: Incorporate Cayenne's fiery presence into your morning rituals. Support your heart by adhering to the guide's principle of loving the morning.

- Culinary Innovation: Try different meals using cayenne. Let the discovery of flavor and nutrition in the guide be echoed by your culinary creativity.

- Mindful Inclusion: When including cayenne in your meals, do it with awareness. Each sprinkle becomes a kind act that reflects the guide's all-encompassing strategy for heart well-being.

- Flavorful Fusion: Blend Cayenne with the previously stated herbs that help the heart for a flavorful fusion. This amalgamation ties in with the guide's investigation of how to combine pieces for a whole-heart melody.

As you include cayenne pepper into your daily routine, keep in mind that every decision you make contributes to the harmony of your heart's health. The incorporation of cayenne into your routine connects with the concept of "Exploring Herbal Approaches for Heart-Health," generating a narrative that embraces both brightness and mindful living, much as herbs mingle to produce harmonious tastes.

7.3 Culinary Flare: Adding Cayenne's Heat to Your Dishes

The intense heat of cayenne pepper is revealed as a transformational ingredient in the world of culinary creation, embodying the guide's all-encompassing investigation of heart fitness. This section, "Culinary Flare: Enriching Your Dishes with Cayenne's Heat," encourages you to do just that, reflecting the guide's emphasis on attentive eating.

- Flavorful Dynamics: Introduce the heat of cayenne to your recipes for a blast of flavor dynamism. Let its searing touch spark a symphony of flavors, reflecting the guide's examination of food.

- Heartfelt Enhancement: Recognize that the presence of cayenne is not simply about heat; rather, it is an enhancer that supports the heart. This concept is consistent with the guide's central idea of using food to promote heart-health.

- Fusion cuisine: Combine Cayenne with a variety of foods to produce delectable tastes. Every combination serves as evidence of the guide's investigation of holistic nutrition.

- Savory Symphony: To give your savory foods a powerful flavor harmony, add cayenne. This echoes the theme of the guide, which is to relish tastes that strengthen the heart.

- Tasteful Transformation: Observe how your foods change when cayenne is added. In keeping with the spirit of the guide, let each mouthful become an investigation of bright flavor.

- **Heart-Healthy Creations:** Create heart-healthy meals by putting cayenne at the forefront. The gastronomic journey of well-being described in the guide is consistent with this culinary inventiveness.

- **Spice with Intention:** Sprinkle Cayenne while being conscious of your aim while you cook. Let each dash represent your dedication to heart wellness, following the guide's all-encompassing philosophy.

- **Fusion of Flavors:** Combine the herbs that assist the heart from earlier with cayenne. This taste fusion complements the guide's investigation of combining ingredients for overall sustenance.

Remember that each meal you create becomes a note in the symphony of your heart's well-being when you add Cayenne's heat to your recipes. The addition of Cayenne to your culinary creations, much as how herbs combine to produce harmonious flavors, fits with the theme of "Exploring Herbal Approaches for Heart-Health," creating a narrative that celebrates both taste and sustenance.

7.4 Cayenne pepper is a spice that may be presented in your meals with finesse.

Cayenne Pepper's hot touch transforms into an artistic stroke within the context of culinary expression, serving as a testament to the guide's all-encompassing exploration of heart fitness. This section, **Spice with Finesse: Presenting Cayenne Pepper in Your Meals**, encourages you to mindfully participate in your culinary experience by skillfully incorporating Cayenne's bright essence into your meals.

- Culinary Elegance: Add Cayenne's fiery elegance to your dishes. Let it add a refined tone to your recipes, complementing the guide's examination of tastes that are good for the heart.

- Vibrant Visuals: Recognize Cayenne's promise for both taste and visual attraction in its vibrant visuals. Its rich color takes on a lively expression, reflecting the guide's focus on sensory stimulation.

Culinary Harmony: Blend cayenne with other substances to create a mellow flavor profile. Let the guide's topic of balanced nutrition be reflected in the symphony of tastes.

- Flavor Sensation: Add Cayenne for a palate-awakening flavor sensation. This is consistent with the guide's advice to deliberately taste flavors that boost the heart.

- Culinary Craftsmanship: Add culinary artistry to Cayenne's essence. The guide's investigation of culinary creativity resonates with how each meal transforms into a painting for heart wellness.

- Presentation with mindfulness: As you dish your food, sprinkle the cayenne pepper with awareness. Let your dedication to heart-health be symbolized by each touch, following the comprehensive philosophy of the guide.

- Fusion of Tastes: Combine Cayenne with the previously stated heart-healthy herbs. Let the mingling of flavors complement the guide's central idea of combining different ingredients to create something wholesome.

- Culinary Expression: Use Cayenne Pepper as the centerpiece of your culinary concept. The investigation of culinary care throughout the guide is consistent with this flavorful presentation.

Remember that any way you arrange Cayenne Pepper in your meals becomes a note in the symphony of your heart-health as you do it with delicacy. The addition of Cayenne Pepper connects with the concept of "Exploring Herbal Approaches for Heart-Health," generating a narrative that embraces both flavor and thoughtful presentation, just as herbs mingle to produce harmonious culinary experiences.

7.5 Timing the Heat: Best Times to Consume Cayenne Pepper

The time of Cayenne Pepper's use emerges as a crucial element within the ebb and flow of daily rhythms, reflecting the guide's comprehensive investigation of heart wellness. In keeping with the guide's idea of conscious engagement, this section, "Timing the Heat: Optimal Moments for Cayenne Pepper Consumption," urges you to time Cayenne's fiery effect with your daily cadence.

- Morning Vitality: Embrace the warmth of Cayenne Pepper in the morning for morning vitality. Its energizing qualities are consistent with the guide's recommendation to use the morning to assist the heart.

- Lunchtime Livening: Add Cayenne's heat to your lunchtime food. In keeping with the guide's topic of sustaining persistent cardiac wellness, let it awaken your senses and nourish your energy.

- Pre-Exercise Boost: Consider taking Cayenne Pepper before working out for a pre-workout boost. Its ability to enhance circulation is consistent with the guide's focus on heart-health while exercising.

- Indulgent Flavor: Add Cayenne's heat to your evening dishes. Make supper a savory indulgence with its presence, complementing the guide's examination of taste and heart-health.

- Mindful Savoring: During meals, combine awareness and cayenne with attentive savoring. The principle of mindful consumption in the guide is mirrored in how each mouthful becomes a time of focused nutrition.

- Heartfelt Rituals: Integrate cayenne pepper into customs like tea time. In keeping with the topic of the guide, use its flaming energy to fill your moments with heart-supporting warmth.

- Holistic Synergy: Combining Cayenne with other heart-healthy substances creates a holistic synergy. Let the guide's discovery of comprehensive harmony in well-being reverberate with the taste combination.

- Culinary Innovation: Try different meals using cayenne. Embrace its fire in your culinary undertakings to complement the guide's emphasis on creative inquiry.

As you keep track of how much cayenne pepper you consume, keep in mind that every decision you make contributes to the harmony of your heart's health. The synchronization of Cayenne with your daily rhythm resonates with the concept of "Exploring Herbal Approaches for Heart-Health," generating a story that embraces both brightness and thoughtful participation, just as herbs mingle to produce harmonious tastes.

7.6 Dosing Cayenne Pepper for Comfort: Finding the Right Heat

The search to discover the proper dosage emerges as a crucial journey during the investigation of Cayenne Pepper's impact on heart wellness—a reflection of the guide's all-encompassing strategy for nourishing the heart. Finding the balance that works for you is encouraged in this part, Finding the Right Heat:

Dosing Cayenne Pepper for Your Comfort, which echoes the guide's emphasis on individualized wellness.

- Personalized Balance: Awareness that your tolerance for cayenne varies. This personalized strategy is consistent with the guide's focus on adjusting cardiac support to your comfort level.

- Sensory Exploration: Cayenne should be included in your regimen gradually. Mirroring the guide's idea of gradual inclusion for well-being, let your body adjust.

- Sensory Investigation: As you take cayenne pepper, pay attention to your senses. Following the principle of mindful feeding advocated in the guide, let your body's response dictate your dose.

- Listen to Your Body: Pay attention to how your body responds to cayenne by listening to it. The signals from your body serve as a compass for regulating your dose, echoing the guide's concept of self-awareness.

- Culinary Creativity: Investigate the various ways you may use cayenne in cooking. Learn how its heat complements different foods, reflecting the guide's research on adaptable cardiac support.

- Gradual Adaptation: Give your body time to adjust. You may follow the guide's advice for heart wellness by gradually increasing your Cayenne consumption.

- Incorporation in Blends: Blending Cayenne with other herbs that assist the heart is a good idea. Let their interaction affect your dose in keeping with the guide's focus on a holistic balance.

- Consultation with Experts: Speak with herbalists or other healthcare providers for advice. Their observations are in line with the guide's recommendation for making educated choices with compassion.

Keep in mind that each change you make to the Cayenne Pepper dosage becomes a note in the harmony of your heart's health as you proceed. The search for the ideal Cayenne dose resonates with the concept of "Exploring Herbal Approaches for Heart-Health," generating a story that emphasizes both customization and holistic treatment, just as herbs mix to produce harmonious tastes.

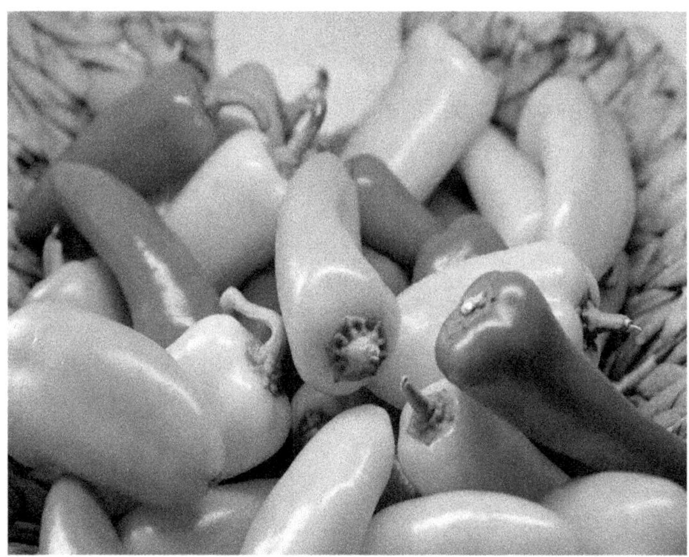

CHAPTER EIGHT: Celery: Crispy Heart Support

8.1 Celery's Crunchy Contribution to Cardiovascular Care

Celery stands out as a clean and energizing note in the symphony of heart wellness, embodying the guide's all-encompassing investigation of herbs for heart-health. In keeping with the natural nutrition ethos of the guide, "Celery: Crispy Heart Support" invites you to taste the special contribution that celery makes to cardiovascular care.

Celery's Dual Nature

The unique dual character of celery as a diuretic and a heart-supportive plant should be embraced. This comprehension is consistent with the guide's central idea—herbs are versatile companions in heart wellness.

Blood Pressure Harmony

Learn about celery's potential for lowering blood pressure. Its phytochemicals complement the guide's examination of herbal support for heart-health by harmoniously relaxing the arterial muscles.

TCM Wisdom

Recognize celery's prestigious status in "Traditional Chinese Medicine (TCM)" as a leading treatment for blood pressure and heart issues. The holistic approach to heart care that the guide takes across multiple traditions is reflected in this alignment.

Negative Calorie Elegance

Explore the elegance of celery's negative calorie nature, which attests to its function in weight loss and energy balance. The emphasis on comprehensive well-being achieved via natural processes is consistent with this throughout the guide.

Sensory Gratification

Enjoy the crunch of celery as a sensory treat. Its sharp texture should reflect the guide's recommendation to interact with herbs tangibly and thoughtfully.

Weight Wellness

Recognize celery's ability to aid with weight management by providing negative-calorie enjoyment. This comprehension is consistent with the guide's holistic health care via nourishing choices concept.

Diverse Preferences

If the flavor of celery doesn't appeal to you, look into substitutes like celery seed extract. This flexible strategy fits with the guide's central idea of personalizing herbal assistance.

Consider how each experience adds to the symphony of your heart's health as you learn more about celery's crisp benefits for heart-health. The addition of celery connects with the concept of "Exploring Herbal Approaches for Heart-Health," generating a story that embraces both taste and overall sustenance, just as plants mingle to create harmonious tastes.

8.2 Easily Including Celery in Your Daily Routine

The technique of seamless blending becomes apparent as you work to include Celery into your lifestyle, reflecting the guide's all-encompassing approach to heart care. The chapter "Blending Celery Seamlessly into Your Daily Regimen" advises you to do just that, using the guide's natural integration concept.

- Daily Integration: Include celery in your routine regularly to help your heart. Allow it to seamlessly integrate into your wellness journey so that it supports the guide's sustainable care idea.

- Culinary Symphonies: Blend the crisp celery with a variety of meals for culinary symphonies. Let it blend in with your culinary creations and echo the examination of balanced nutrition in the guide.

- Snack Sensibility: Accept celery as a heart-healthy snack. In keeping with the conscious consuming ethos of the guide, its sharpness is transformed into a thoughtful pleasure.

- Fluid Fusion: Add celery to your smoothies or fresh juices. As a reflection of the emphasis on holistic nourishment throughout the guide, observe the confluence of tastes and nutrients.

- Pairings for the Plate: Combine celery with other items that are good for the heart. Let your devotion to well-being be symbolized by their combination, following the holistic healthcare concept of the guide.

- Inventive Modifications: Experiment with celery in other cuisines. Let your imagination guide you, in keeping with the guide's examination of adaptable cardiac support.

- Mindful Eating: Savor your Celery with awareness while you eat. Each mouthful transforms into a heart-stirring moment of awareness, embodying the idea of the guide.

- Customized Options: Tailor your consumption of celery to your tastes. This personalized strategy supports the guide's recommendation for individualized cardiac support.

Remember that when you incorporate Celery into your routine, each action adds a note to the harmony of your heart's health. The integration of celery connects with the concept of "Exploring Herbal Approaches for Heart-Health," generating a story that embraces both taste and natural fusion. Herbs unite to create harmonious tastes in much the same way.

8.3 Culinary Harmony: Infusing Fresh Celery Into Your Meals"

Celery's freshness creates a harmonizing chord in the world of culinary expression, a witness to the guide's all-encompassing investigation of cardiac fitness. The guide's philosophy of mindful nutrition, "Culinary Harmony: Infusing Your Meals with Celery's Freshness" advises you to infuse celery's vitality into your recipes.

- Vibrant Integration: Integrate Celery's lively presence into your dishes with ease by using the vibrant integration technique. Let the guide's subject of balanced nutrition resonate with its freshness as it naturally becomes a part of your culinary symphony.

- Flavorful Fusion: Blend a variety of ingredients with celery's mild flavor for a flavorful fusion. Let its flavor blend with others, reflecting the guide's examination of many forms of cardiac care.

- Sensory Indulgence: Enjoy the crunchy snap of the celery as a sensory treat. Enjoy the sensory sensation as you include it in your meals to support the guide's focus on mindful consumption.

- Culinary Elegance: Use Celery's aesthetic and gustatory elegance to elevate your recipes. Let the freshness of this ingredient enhance your culinary creations as the guide's examination of heart-healthy tastes does.

- Balanced Compositions: Create dishes with balanced compositions by including celery. Let the freshness blend with the other components in keeping with the overall well-being idea of the guide.

- Culinary Exploration: Investigate the use of celery in diverse cuisines via experimentation. Allow the guide's appeal for imaginative inquiry to resonate with its freshness as it adds a dimension of culinary adventure.

- Mindful Presentation: Plate your meals with celery's presence in mind for a thoughtful presentation. Regarding the guide's concept of deliberate consumption, its freshness becomes a focal point of heart nutrition.

- Visual Delight: Recognize how celery's green color enhances the aesthetic appeal of your food. Its existence is consistent with the guide's focus on sensory fulfillment as heart support.

Remember that when you include the freshness of celery into your culinary creations, each addition becomes a note in the harmony of your heart's health. The integration of celery connects with the concept of "Exploring Herbal Approaches for Heart-Health," generating a story that honors both taste and deliberate culinary expression, just as herbs mingle to create harmonious sensations.

8.4 Serving Crispness: How to Highlight the Health Benefits of Celery"

A symphony of serving options emerges in the art of presenting Celery's advantages, reflecting the guide's all-encompassing approach to heart care. As a nod to the guide's idea of attentive involvement, "Serving Crispness: Ways to Present Celery's Benefits" asks you to highlight Celery's benefits in a variety of ways.

- **Fresh Snacking:** Provide celery as a crunchy and revitalizing snack. Its simplicity serves as evidence for the emphasis on natural food throughout the guide.

- **Salad Sensation:** Celery may provide crispness to salads, according to Salad Sensation. As the guide explores balanced heart support, let its presence enrich your salad creations.

- **Heartfelt Hydration:** Add celery to water that has been infused. Witness how its presence echoes the guide's concept of comprehensive care by infusing your hydration with heart-supporting freshness.

- **Culinary Garnish:** Celery may be used as a garnish on several foods. Its aesthetic appeal and flavor complement the guide's examination of sensory fulfillment in heart fitness.

- Smoothie Booster: Blend celery into your smoothies for a boost. Its sharpness adds to the texture and flavor in keeping with the guide's emphasis on nourishing the heart in a variety of ways.

- Culinary Medley: Celery should be included in stir-fries and sautés. Let its crunchiness accentuate the mix of tastes, evoking the notion of all-encompassing harmony found in the guide.

- Appetizer Extravaganza: Present celery sticks as an appetizer in this extravaganza of an appetizer. Its simplicity transforms into a delectable introduction to heart-healthy meals, mirroring the spirit of the guide.

- Fresh Juice Infusion: Celery may be infused into fresh juices by doing so. Watch how, like the guide's appeal for attentive consumption, its essence becomes a part of your everyday routine.

Remember that each presentation becomes a note in the symphony of your heart's well-being as you consider approaches to serve Celery's advantages. The highlighting of celery connects with the concept of "Exploring Herbal Approaches for Heart-Health," generating a story that honors both flavor and artistic expression, much as herbs combine to produce harmonious tastes.

8.5 Time for Freshness: Choosing the Appropriate Times for Celery

Finding the right times to use celery develops in the rhythm of heart care, reflecting the guide's all-encompassing approach to herbal assistance. In keeping with the guide's idea of mindful feeding, "Time for Freshness: Identifying the Right Times for Celery" urges you to determine when the freshness of celery corresponds with your daily schedule.

- Morning Awakening: Start your day with the fresh vigor of celery. Your daily routine will be given a fresh start as a result, complementing the guide's examination of comprehensive well-being.

- **Midday Refreshment:** Include celery as a noon snack with your midday meal. In keeping with the notion of balanced nourishment throughout the guide, let its crunch revitalize your energies.

- **Pre-Meal Prelude:** Eat celery before meals as a prelude. Its freshness transforms into a savory introduction to foods that are heart-nourishing, in keeping with the guide's emphasis on deliberate eating.

- **Hydration Breaks:** Utilize celery in your regimen for hydration breaks. Observe how it improves your water intake as a nod to the guide's subject of all-encompassing care.

- **Post-Workout Refueling:** Savor Celery's advantages following the exercise. Its energizing crunch compliments your post-workout routine and embodies the guide's emphasis on total wellness.

- **Cooking Companion:** Include celery in your meals. Let it enhance your meals as the guide explores the versatility of cardiac support.

- Evening Farewell: End your day with the crispness of celery. In keeping with the guide's premise, its inclusion becomes a calming tone in your nightly routines.

- **Mindful Pause:** Pause mindfully and pay attention to your body's cues. Recognize the moments when Celery's sharpness corresponds with your body's need, in keeping with the guide's focus on self-awareness.

Remember that each moment becomes a note in the symphony of your heart's well-being as you decide when Celery should be included. The timing of celery connects with the spirit of "Exploring Herbal Approaches for Heart-Health," generating a story that emphasizes both time and attentive participation, just as herbs combine to create harmonious tastes.

8.6 Balancing Green Goodness: Determining Your Celery Dosage

Determining your Celery dose takes on a new meaning in the world of green wellness as a reflection of the guide's all-encompassing approach to heart-health. In keeping with the guide's emphasis on mindful eating, this section, "Balancing Green Goodness: Determining Your Celery Dosage," urges you to find your balance when it comes to celery consumption.

- Personalized Alignment: Pay attention to your body's cues to determine the right Celery dose. Follow your body's demands, just as the guide explores customized cardiac care.

- Gradual Integration: Begin with a moderate intake of celery and increase it over time. In keeping with the guide's premise of progressive, sustained care, let your body adjust.

- Observational Method: Pay attention to how your body reacts to celery. Consider your observations while choosing your dose, keeping in mind the guide's focus on self-awareness.

- Culinary Exploration: Investigate many meals that contain celery in the kitchen. Your dose decisions should be influenced by your culinary investigation, in keeping with the guide's emphasis on creative participation.

- Consultative Actions: Ask a medical expert for advice. Talk about your celery intake and heart-health objectives to achieve the best dose, in keeping with the guide's emphasis on holistic cooperation.

- Holistic Integration: Integrate celery into many elements of your routine for holistic integration. Let its presence resonate with the guide's investigation of total health support and become a part of your entire well-being.

- Taste and Preference: Let your dose be determined by your taste preferences. Embrace celery in ways that suit your palette, keeping with the personalized care ethos of the guide.

- Conscious Modification: Regularly reevaluate your celery dose. Let your path be one of thoughtful changes, following the guide's advice to maintain heart support that is attentive and continual.

Keep in mind that every modification you make to your Celery dose becomes a note in the symphony of your heart's health. The dose of celery connects with the concept of "Exploring Herbal Approaches for Heart-Health," generating a story that emphasizes both balance and attentive participation, just as herbs combine to produce harmonious tastes.

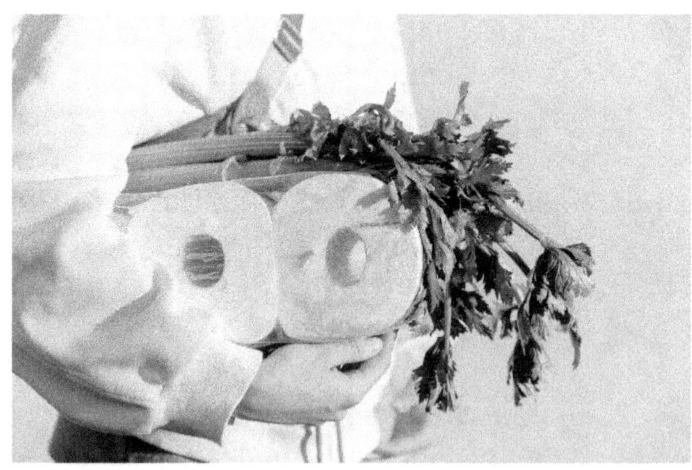

CHAPTER NINE: Garlic: A Flavorful Shield for the Heart

The symphony of heart support that develops in the fragrant embrace of garlic's health benefits serves as evidence of the guide's comprehensive approach to cardiovascular health. "Garlic: A Flavorful Shield for the Heart" investigates the important impacts of garlic's aromatic essence on your circulatory vitality, in keeping with the herbal study topic of the title.

9.1: The Aromatic Effects of Garlic on Cardiovascular Health

The versatility of garlic reveals itself as a heart-friendly friend. Garlic has some advantages and is a superb safeguard. It is masterful at reducing cholesterol and improving blood thickness for more fluid flow. Its benefits also include moderate hypertension since it helps reduce blood pressure. The harmonious combination of garlic and your blood clotting ability results in a symphony of health. The order in which these attributes are presented reflects the focus placed in the guidance on overall heart health.

The Simplicity of Consumption

It's amazing how easily accessible garlic is; no complicated rituals are needed. Make liberal use of it in your culinary creations to let the essence blend with the tastes. Alternately, practice a daily routine that involves consuming a tablespoon of chopped garlic mixed with a little bit of honey. The straightforwardness of this strategy represents the guide's simple and common-sense approach to cardiac support.

Aromatic Essences and Herbal Integration

Although garlic's flavor doesn't exactly go with tea, its adaptability in the kitchen makes a variety of meals taste better. Its fragrant brightness goes well with savory dishes, reflecting the guide's investigation of flavor-filled heart nourishment.

The Flavorful Guardian of the Heart

Consider garlic to be your savory protector and friend for the health of your heart. Garlic's inclusion connects with the guide's theme of holistic nutrition, just as herbs combine to create mellow tastes.

Talking to Health Care Professionals

Before making large modifications, it is wise to consult healthcare specialists, as with any herb. The emphasis on cooperative cardiac care in the guide is consistent with having open discussions.

Culinary Synergy

Include garlic in your regular meals so that other components can benefit from its fragrant overtones. The fragrant influence of garlic, which is used to flavor food, parallels the guide's appeal for overall heart-health.

Remember that each experience you have as you explore the fragrant world of garlic's health benefits adds a note to the harmony of your heart's well-being. The addition of Garlic connects with the concept of "Exploring Herbal Approaches for Heart-Health," generating a narrative that embraces both taste and attentive participation, just as herbs mingle to create harmonious tastes.

9.2 Incorporating the Essence of Garlic Into Your Daily Routine

Garlic's essence is woven into the fabric of daily activities, reflecting the guide's all-encompassing approach to heart-health. In keeping with the guide's premise of easily accessible nutrition, "Infusing Garlic's Essence into Your Daily Routine" urges you to smoothly absorb Garlic's advantages.

- Culinary Symphony: Increase the quality of your meals by cooking with garlic. Its fragrant undertones blend beautifully with the guide's examination of flavor-rich cardiac care.

- Savory Improvements: Use garlic to add flavor to food. Let its fragrant allure enhance the tastes of your foods, reflecting the guide's emphasis on all-encompassing heart care.

- Nutritious Ritual: Adopt the practice of eating a tablespoon of honey and chopped garlic every day. In keeping with the guide's concept of attainable heart well-being, experience its simplicity and ease.

- Flavorsome Allies: This combines garlic with other heart-healthy foods. Watch how its essence blends with other flavors to create a harmonious culinary experience, mirroring the guide's concept.

- Artistry in the kitchen: Examine the use of garlic in various recipes. Accept its core as a work of culinary artistry that echoes the guide's exhortation to use creativity to promote heart-health.

- Daily Enrichment: Include garlic in a number of your meals each day. Let its fragrant flavor provide depth to your culinary creations, echoing the guide's discussion of regular nutrition.

- Palate harmony: Incorporate garlic into foods that suit your palette. Take in its essence in ways that suit your palate, matching the guide's emphasis on individualized heart care.

- Culinary Interest: Play around with garlic Allow your culinary curiosity to lead you, following the guide's guiding principle of ongoing investigation into heart-health.

Remember that each time you incorporate the essence of garlic into your daily routine, it adds a new note to the harmonious melody of your heart's health. The addition of Garlic connects with the concept of "Exploring Herbal Approaches for Heart-Health," generating a story that embraces both routine and thoughtful participation, just as herbs mingle to produce harmonious tastes.

9.3 Culinary Fusions: Using the Aroma of Garlic to Improve Your Recipes"

Garlic's perfume emerges amid the culinary artistry as a representation of the guide's all-inclusive approach to heart-health. The guide's motto, "Flavor-Enriched Nutrition," is echoed in the invitation to embrace garlic's fragrant essence in Culinary Fusions: Enhancing Your Recipes with Garlic's Aroma".

- Aromatic Symphony: Allows the scent of garlic to complement your food. As the guide explores complete cardiac support, let its fragrant notes create an olfactory symphony.

- Flair-Adding Accents: Use the fragrant accents of garlic to elevate your meals. Watch how the perfume enhances the taste sensation, echoing the guide's focus on improving heart wellness.

- Culinary Inspiration: Inspiration for Food Utilize the fragrant power of garlic in your cooking. In keeping with the guide's concept of culinary discovery for heart-health, including its scent in a variety of dishes.

- Savory Infusions: Include the flavor of garlic in dressings, marinades, and sauces. Discover how the guide's thematic focus on different heart support is echoed by the way its fragrance infusion improves the delicious appeal.

- Aromatic Relationships: Combine the flavor of the garlic with supplementary herbs and spices. See for yourself how their complementary aromas enhance the richness of flavors, echoing the guide's emphasis on holistic culinary harmony.

- **Everyday Aroma:** Make Garlic's scent a staple by adding it frequently. Let its perfume accompany you on all your culinary experiences, as the guide encourages ongoing fragrant involvement.

- **Palate Enchantment:** Adjust the scent of garlic to your palate's preferences. Use its olfactory enchantment to your taste, matching the guide's emphasis on individualized heart feeding.

- **Aroma Exploration:** Examine the plethora of flavors that garlic has to offer. In line with the guide's emphasis on ongoing culinary inquiry, let your culinary experimentation reveal its fragrant potential.

As you add the pungent essence of garlic to your meals, keep in mind that each dish you make contributes a note to the harmony of your heart's health. The perfume of garlic is infused with the spirit of "Exploring Herbal Approaches for Heart-Health," creating a story that embraces both taste and attentive participation, much as herbs combine to create harmonious tastes.

9.4 Serving Savory: Showcasing Garlic's Role in Your Dishes

Garlic is the star of the culinary show, demonstrating the guide's all-encompassing approach to heart care. The guide's idea of flavor-rich nutrition is echoed in "Serving Savory: Highlighting Garlic's Role in Your Dishes", which puts attention on garlic's crucial significance.

- Culinary Highlights: Allow garlic to shine in your meals. Its presence becomes the guide's main focus as it examines comprehensive cardiac care.

- Accentuation with flavor: Use garlic to add taste by accentuating it. Observe how it enhances the flavor experience, aligning with the focus of the guide on enhancing food for heart-health.

- Integration through food: Integrate garlic easily into a variety of cuisines. Let it play a part in many culinary customs, in keeping with the guide's subject of flexible culinary exploration.

- Savory Transformations: Watch how using garlic in your food can improve a dish. It contributes to the guide's theme of varied and comprehensive heart feeding as it conveys its meaning.

- Palate Complements: Combine garlic with foods that enhance its wonderful flavor. Discover how it complements other flavors, mirroring the guide's guiding principle of gastronomic friendship for heart support.

- Daily Presence: Make sure you always include garlic in your dishes. In keeping with the guide's advice for consistent and tasty participation, let its role become a part of your regular cooking experiences.

- Personalized Palate: Adjust Garlic's function to your tastes. Accept its flavor in ways that suit your taste buds, in keeping with the guide's emphasis on individualized heart nutrition.

- Culinary Investigation: Take up the role of Garlic and go off on a gastronomic exploration. Allow your culinary explorations to reveal its numerous functions, echoing the guide's emphasis on ongoing culinary exploration.

Remember that each culinary creation becomes a note in the symphony of your heart's well-being as you offer the savory essence of garlic in your meals. Garlic's position in your recipes connects with the concept of "Exploring Herbal Approaches for Heart-Health," generating a narrative that celebrates both taste and attentive participation, just as herbs combine to produce harmonious tastes.

9.5 Timing the Flavor: Best Times to Enjoy the Goodness of Garlic"

The timing of Garlic's appearance within the cadence of culinary discovery is crucial—a reflection of the guide's all-inclusive approach to heart care. The chapter "Timing the Flavor: Optimal Times to Enjoy Garlic's Goodness" echoes the guide's emphasis on attentive eating by guiding you through the best times to appreciate garlic's deliciousness.

- Morning Vitality: Infuse the essence of garlic into your breakfast to start the day. Like the guide's examination of holistic heart support, let its presence give your day a savory lift.

- Midday Restoration: Include the taste of garlic in your lunchtime dishes. As the guide emphasizes constant heart nutrition, see how its goodness awakens your senses and sustains your vitality.

- Afternoon uplift: Include the benefits of garlic in your afternoon snacks and meals. Observe how its presence enhances your palate and energy levels, echoing the subject of comprehensive heart care throughout the guide.

- Afternoon Indulgence: Include garlic in your evening's indulgent meals. Let its flavor enhance your dinners, connecting with the guide's emphasis on heart wellness all day long.

- Gastronomic Symmetry: Combine the flavors of garlic with foods that enhance its taste. Observe how the timing echoes the idea of the guide, which emphasizes the nutrition of the harmonious heart.

- Culinary Investigation: Play around with the timing of the garlic in different dishes. In keeping with the guide's emphasis on ongoing research in heart fitness, let your appetite choose the occasions when it shines.

- Personal Palate: Adjust the time of the garlic to your taste preferences. Enjoy its flavor when it suits your palate, in keeping with the guide's emphasis on individualized heart nutrition.

- Reflective Periods: Use the flavor of garlic when you want to ponder or unwind. Your culinary experiences should be improved by its presence, echoing the guide's call for thoughtful involvement in heart support.

Keep in mind that each time you enjoy the flavor of garlic, it adds a new note to the harmony of your heart's health. The timing of garlic's goodness connects with the essence of "Exploring Herbal Approaches for

Heart-Health," generating a narrative that celebrates both time and attentive participation, just as herbs combine to create harmonious tastes.

9.6 Measuring Aroma: Selecting the Appropriate Garlic Dosage

Finding the perfect balance of garlic's scent becomes crucial within the tapestry of culinary discovery, reflecting the guide's all-encompassing viewpoint on heart-health. As part of the guide's philosophy of balanced nutrition, "Gauging the Aroma: Determining the Right Garlic Dosage" enables you to determine the optimal dosage of garlic's essence.

- Culinary equilibrium: Try to balance the odor of garlic with your food. Let it complement, not dominate, the examination of comprehensive cardiac care in the guide.

- Flavorsome Harmony: Harmoniously combine various flavors with the fragrance of garlic. Discover how the dose harmonizes with the entire flavor, echoing the guide's focus on complete heart nutrition.

- Incremental Investigation: Start with a small amount of the garlic fragrance. Reflecting on the subject of the guide's cautious and thoughtful heart support, observe its effects and gradually make adjustments.

- Culinary Cooperation: Include the scent of garlic in a variety of meals. The guide's emphasis on comprehensive culinary friendship is echoed by the way its dose works with diverse foods.

- Palate Alignment: Adjust the dose of garlic to suit your palate's preferences. Its scent should be embraced in quantities that suit your preferences, representing the guide's individualized approach to heart care.

- Culinary Curiosity: Try out different dose amounts. In keeping with the guide's emphasis on the ongoing discovery of heart nutrition, let your appetite lead you.

- Reflective Engagement: Analyze how the smell of garlic affects your health. In keeping with the guide's recommendation for balanced and considerate heart support, let its dose become a part of your attentive culinary interaction.

- **Aromatic Presence:** Accept the fragrance of garlic as a useful complement. Choose the dose that best emphasizes the herb's fragrant presence while also reflecting the guide's theme of thoughtful and balanced heartfeeding.

Remember that each culinary venture becomes a note in the symphony of your heart's well-being as you choose the proper quantity of garlic's fragrance. The ideal amount of garlic's essence resonates with the essence of "Exploring Herbal Approaches for Heart-Health," generating a narrative that celebrates both proportion and attentive participation, just as herbs mingle to create harmonious tastes.

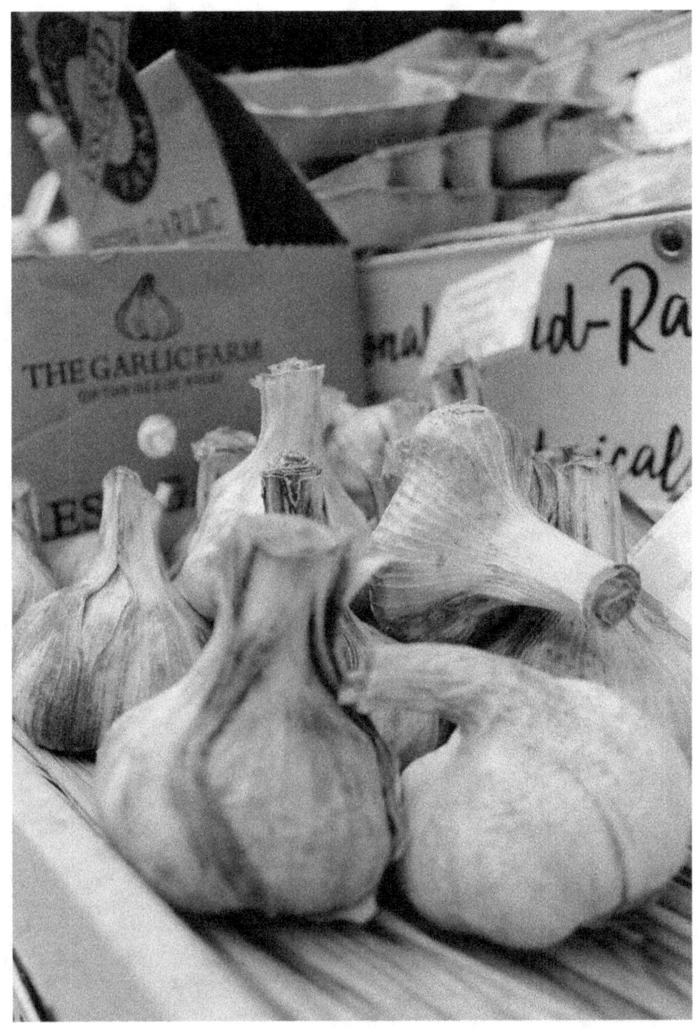
THE GARLIC FARM

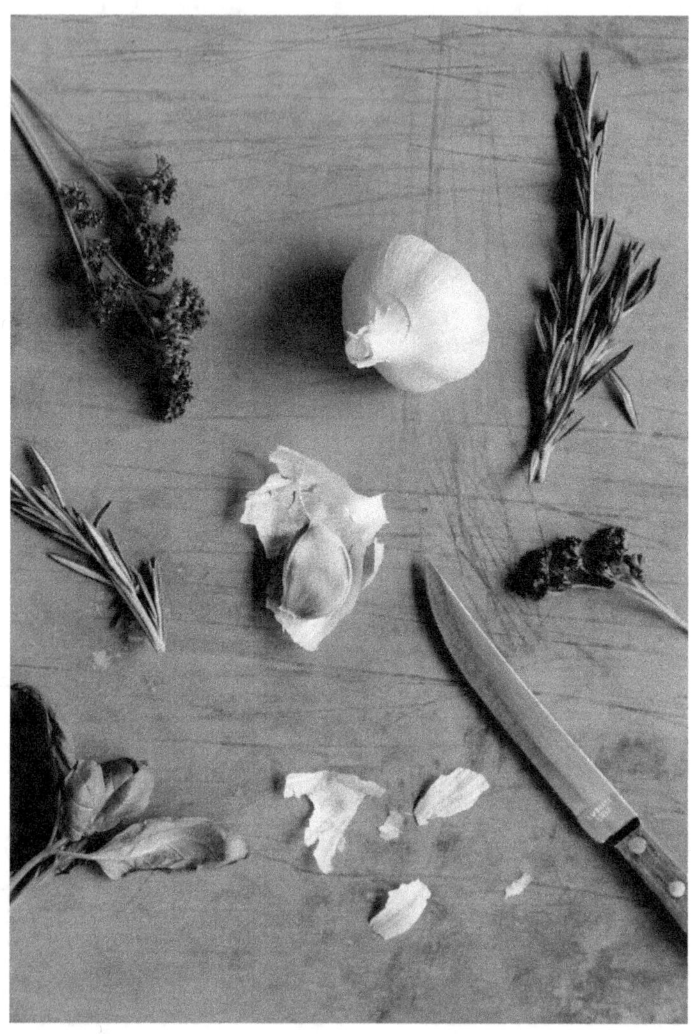

CHAPTER TEN: Serving Savory: Highlighting Garlic's Role in Your Dishes

The unfolding of Chapter 10—a mellow continuation of the herbal symphony that comes before it—takes place in the center of the gastronomic investigation. As the conclusion of our trip, "Serving Savory: Highlighting Garlic's Role in Your Dishes" emerges as a reminder that heart fitness is a tasty and interesting endeavor, deeply woven into daily life.

10.1 Making a Personalized Herbal Plan for Heart Wellness

Garlic comes forward to grace our dishes and palates as we review the herbs we traveled with from Chapter 2 to Chapter 9. The focus of the guide's last chapter, however, is not simply on garlic; rather, it is on combining all the knowledge into a unique plan for heart wellness that captures the spirit of the guide's all-encompassing philosophy.

Reflection on Our Herbal Path

Every plant, including hibiscus, hawthorn, rooibos, motherwort, ginger, cayenne pepper, and celery, has contributed a special note to our understanding of heart-health. Each chapter echoes the symphony they jointly create, and the conclusion, Garlic, captures the coherence of their efforts.

Creating Your Herbal Symphony

Think about the unique characteristics of each herb as you go toward developing a specialized herbal plan for heart fitness. Every herb contributes to the health of your heart in the same way as each instrument does in a symphony. Consider your tastes, requirements, and lifestyle when selecting your herbs to reflect the guide's focus on individualized treatment.

Herbal Harmony in Culinary Creations

Your culinary journey will parallel the story of this guide, from sipping Hibiscus tea to enjoying garlic-infused foods. The incorporation of these herbs into your meals corresponds with the guide's theory of culinary harmony, just as in a symphony, where melodies blend to produce lovely harmonies.

Nourishment Beyond Taste

Each herb delivers a variety of heart-supporting advantages in addition to flavor. The holistic perspective of the guide is embodied by the vasodilating effects of hawthorn, the relaxing embrace of motherwort, and the fiery vigor of cayenne pepper. Together, they provide a symphony of well-being that enhances your path toward better heart-health.

A Strategy for Daily Life

Accept these plants into your daily life as partners rather than as ingredients. Your unique herbal plan delivers continual heart support, much as a symphony uplifts and comforts. Let this plan serve as a daily reminder of your dedication to heart fitness, from the refreshing drink of Hibiscus to the perfume of Garlic's embrace.

Consultative Steps

Engage healthcare providers in talks as you're finalizing your plan. Your road toward better heart-health benefits from collaborative assistance, much as a conductor does when looking for experienced musicians' suggestions. Accept the knowledge of both herbal and medical knowledge, reflecting the emphasis on all-encompassing care in the guide.

Crafting a Heart-Centered Lifestyle

In the end, this chapter is about more than simply garlic; it's about developing a heart-centered lifestyle, one that is motivated by the plants that have adorned our path. Your heart-centered lifestyle weaves stories of nutrition, energy, and well-being, much as a symphony conveys emotions and narratives.

A Culmination of Flavors and Wisdom

Chapter 10 is the culmination of our voyage through the herbal symphony; it is a tapestry of tastes and insights that form the core of your well-being. May the essence of these plants stay in your heart, echoing with the spirit of "Exploring Herbal Approaches for Health," much as the last note of a symphony does.

10.2   Integrating   Herbs   into Lifestyle Choices

The skill of balancing herbal remedies with lifestyle decisions—a complex ballet that orchestrates holistic heart-health—is at the center of this guide. The symphony of herbs blended with the rhythms of daily life as we read through the chapters, creating a route to well-being.

- Incorporating synergistically: The herbs easily fit into our habits, much as how musical notes meld to form harmonies. Each herb creates a story that highlights the connection between herbal treatments and way of life choices by resonating with our everyday lives.

- Reflective Balance: We establish equilibrium in our decisions, much as a conductor balances tunes. From Hibiscus to Garlic, the plants offered knowledge and sustenance, reflecting the balance desired for heart wellness.

- Carefully Constructed: We deliberately designed our approach to heart-health, much like a symphony. Herbal infusions, delectable dishes, and thoughtful dosing were deliberate choices that echoed the emphasis on attentive interaction in the guide.

- Melodies of Wellness: The same way a symphony stirs up feelings, the herbs do the same. Every swig of hibiscus tea and every sprinkling of cayenne pepper resounded with the promise of a heart that was healthier—a tune written by botanical knowledge.

- Holistic resonance: The core of the guide reverberated in heart-centered life, much like a symphony does throughout a room. Every plant, from the soothing hug of hawthorn to the zesty jolt of ginger, embodied the overall philosophy of the guide.

- Living Peaceably: Our adventure inspired us to live in harmony, just the way musicians practice to develop their harmony. The herbs instructed us on how to combine food with purpose, mirroring the guide's admonition for living from the heart.

- Nourishment and sustenance: The plants nurture the heart in the same manner as a symphony that nourishes the spirit. According to the guide's premise, each plant provided sustenance, from the calming sips of Rooibos to the fragrant hug of garlic.

- Developing Vitality: Our interaction with the herbs cultivates vitality inside ourselves, much like listening to a symphony does for its audience. The plants cultivated heart wellness and echoed the idea of the guide as they entwined with our lives.

The blending of herbs and lifestyle decisions produces a melody of heart well-being in the symphony of life. The trip through "Exploring Herbal Approaches for Heart-Health" leaves us with a symphony of energy, reverberating in the decisions we make for our hearts, just like music offers delight to the soul.

10.3 Choosing Doses and Frequency"

The management of doses and frequency emerged as a critical component throughout our investigation of herbal treatments for heart-health—a complicated choreography that directs our wellness path.

- Dosage as Accuracy: It takes accuracy to determine the proper amount, much like when tuning an instrument. Every herb, whether it is hibiscus or motherwort, requires a specific strategy, in line with the focus of the guide on individualized care.

- Harmonizing Frequencies: Similar to how rhythm is important in music, frequency is important in the rhythm of herbal use. Like the pulse of a tune, consistency is essential. Regular use of the herbs is consistent with the guide's idea of continual participation.

- Holistic Integration: Our holistic approach integrates medicines and lifestyle choices, much like a musical group does with different instruments. In keeping with the general principle of the guide, dosages, and frequencies are smoothly incorporated into our regular activities.

- Equitable Practice: We achieve balance in dose and frequency, much as musicians rehearse for balance. The herbs provide a balanced practice that mirrors the guide's emphasis on harmony when taken in moderation at strategic intervals.

- Individual Symphony: Every person's road to wellness necessitates a unique symphony of doses and frequencies, just as every musical composition has a unique beat. Herbal medicines that are carefully selected and used have a place in this unique mixture.

- Sustained Engagement: Consistent doses and frequency keep us interested in herbal therapies, just like a musical score does. When used regularly, herbs become an essential component of our heart-centered way of living.

- Dynamic Modifications: We dynamically alter doses and frequencies in response to our changing demands, just like a conductor alters pace. This responsiveness demonstrates how the guide promotes methods for adaptable well-being.

- Insightful Results: Similar to how music evokes emotions in listeners, the correct doses and frequencies produce heartfelt outcomes. When dosed and ingested thoughtfully, the herbs mimic the heart-focused effects described in the guide, including decreased blood pressure and improved circulation.

Our journey through "Exploring Herbal Approaches for Heart-Health" develops a rhythm as we harmonize doses and frequencies—a cadence of well-being, resonance, and nourished vitality. Our interaction with herbs affects our heart's health, creating a symphony of well-being, just like music transforms environments.

10.4 Savoring a Heart-Centered Lifestyle: Your Path Forward"

The future is revealed in the tapestry of our investigation into herbal treatments for heart-health; this future begs us to relish a heart-centered lifestyle, full of sustenance and intention.

- The pinnacle of wisdom: Our journey through herbs comes to an end with knowledge, much like the last note in a musical composition. From Hibiscus to Garlic, each chapter has contributed valuable insights into the harmony of heart wellness.

- Empowered Decisions: Your path entails making empowered decisions, just like a musician choosing notes with care. The qualities and advantages of the herbs have given you the power to select a way of life that is in harmony with the health of your heart.

- Daily Rhythms: These herbs are now a part of your everyday rhythms, much like the cadence of music. The emphasis on rhythm throughout the guide is reflected in the way that infusions, culinary fusions, and careful dosing meld into the song of your well-being.

- Heart-centered Intention: Your heart-centered lifestyle expresses intention, just as music does. You give heart-health a purpose with each meal and sip, perfectly integrating it with the story's heart-centered theme.

- Consistent Harmony: Your heart-centered lifestyle conveys the harmonies of herbs, just as a symphony contains melodies. The herbs continue to blend inside of you, from the calming Hibiscus tea to the energizing Ginger.

- Lifelong Symphony: The herbs accompany your lifelong path toward healing in the same way that music does. Your life's chapters will be infused with their heart-healthy tunes, mirroring the guide's emphasis on longevity.

- Individualized Score: Your heart-centered lifestyle is a customized score, much like a composer who writes music for a particular audience. It embodies the appeal of the unconventional ways described in the guide and is made with herbs, nutrition, and intention.

- Bright Reflection: Your heart-centered decisions create a bright reflection, similar to how music leaves a lingering resonance. Herb-infused well-being becomes a reflection of your mindful lifestyle thanks to your devotion to it.

The way forward is one of savoring—of a heart-centered life that combines wisdom with intention, wisdom with choices, and herbs. May the echoes of this voyage stay in your heart, guiding you along the peaceful road you've chosen, just as the echoes of music do.

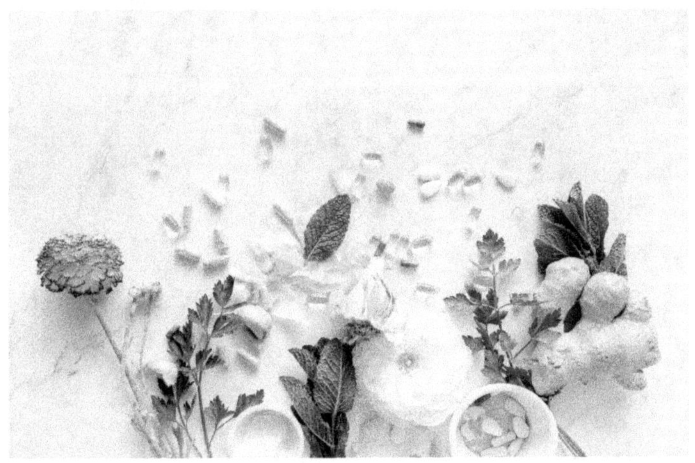

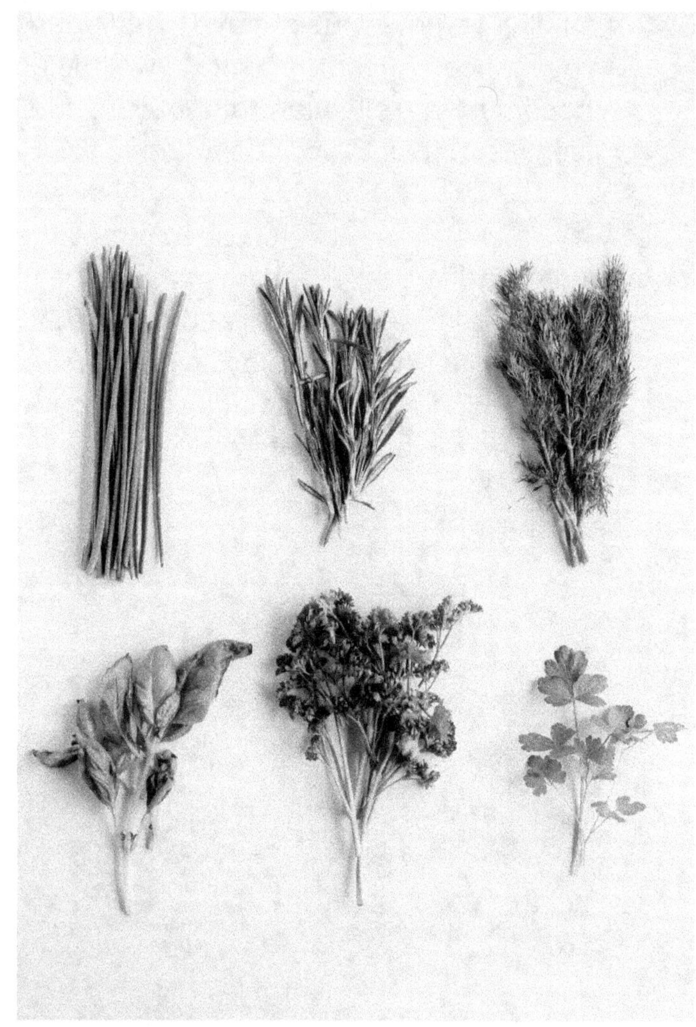

CONCLUSION

Adopting a Holistic Approach to heart-health

As we put the finishing touches on our exploration of herbal heart support, we find ourselves in a state of introspection, comprehension, and continued dedication to our cardiovascular health. Herbal harmony combined with lifestyle decisions has produced a heart-centered living story that speaks to us on a deep level.

Reflecting on Your Journey Through Herbal Heart Support

We learned at the outset of our trip that heart-health is a comprehensive journey, not simply a goal. We discovered the power of plants like Hibiscus, Hawthorn, Rooibos, Motherwort, Ginger, Cayenne Pepper, Celery, and Garlic, each of which contributed a distinctive note to the composition of the life of our hearts. The chapters played out like musical compositions, with each note adding to the overall wellness theme.

We developed the ability to dance in unison with the herbs, much like a conductor leading his symphony, through careful doses and frequencies. Our everyday lives were improved by the culinary use of herbs, which gave our food taste and nutrition.The artful presentation of herbs transformed ordinary circumstances into heart-nourishing moments. Consumption time, used as a metronome, assisted us in determining the rhythm of the greatest advantages.

The Continuous Commitment to Your Cardiovascular Wellness

The road toward the harmony of our hearts is still ongoing; it has not reached its conclusion. The lessons we've learned from the herbs are still relevant today and have a positive impact on the way we live. The knowledge of the herbs resonates in our deliberate decisions, just like a tune does.

The key to holistic heart-health is adopting a way of life that feeds both the body and the soul, not simply the herbs themselves. It has to do with the decisions we make when we eat, the awareness we bring to every herbal tea we drink, and the intention we put into our health routines.

We go on with a fresh sense of agency and empowerment as we get to the end of our exploration. Our knowledge of how to create a song for heart wellness that melds seamlessly with the beat of our life is a gift from the symphony of herbs. We renew our dedication to providing the most comprehensive and meaningful care for our hearts with each sip, nibble, and herb-infused moment.

The trip through "Exploring Herbal Approaches for Heart-Health" is a precursor to a life filled with the melodies of heart-centered living rather than its conclusion. May our hearts echo with the symphony of herbs and decisions, creating a life of energy, well-being, and thriving cardiovascular health, just as a symphony moves its listeners.